'A remarkable book by a remarkable m̶ ... ̶t
of the AIDS epidemic in South A̶ ... ̶n
yet with the balance which is t̶o̶ ... ̶
juc̶
Sydney Ke̶ ...

'If truth is beauty, this relentlessl̶ ... ̶nt and hopeful book is
beautiful. It is a text to live by, if we aspire to the possibility of a
better life for all...in a world widely threatened by HIV/Aids.'
Nadine Gordimer, Nobel Laureate for Literature

'A compelling, principled, and compassionate account of a
remarkable South African's humanitarian quest for responses
to the HIV AIDS pandemic which are scientifically and
constitutionally well-founded.'
John Hood, Vice-Chancellor of Oxford University

'Edwin Cameron's book is important for all who want insight into
the impact of AIDS on our world. Its portrayal of living with HIV
is devastatingly honest – but it also inspires hope, because we
have power to change the conditions of many millions in Africa
and elsewhere who face death in the epidemic.'
Elton John, chairman and founder,
Elton John AIDS Foundation

'Compassionate, passionate, courageous and compelling...'
Shaun Johnson, CEO, Mandela Rhodes Foundation

'Edwin Cameron is a very brave man; and this is a brave, honest,
and uplifting book. A prominent human rights lawyer and
outstanding judge, his pioneering decision to stand up and say
that he was living with HIV is captured here in all its turmoil and
all its pride. It's a moving story, brilliantly told.'
Chris Smith, former Secretary of State for Culture

'The HIV/AIDS epidemic has produced a few thoughtful and
quiet heroes. Judge Edwin Cameron is one of them. His thought-
provoking memoir is a breathtakingly beautiful story of our times.'
Susan Hunter, independent consultant,
UNAIDS, UNICEF and USAID

'I love being a judge. The challenges are exhilarating ... But I am not only a judge. I am also living with AIDS. I am still the only public office bearer in South Africa to have chosen to make public my HIV status. I felt I was called to witness. I felt called to account for my survival in a country in which hundreds of thousands were dying. I did not feel I should remain silent.'

When Edwin Cameron announced to a stunned local and international media that he – one of South Africa's most prominent citizens – was himself living with the virus cutting swathes through the population of the continent, the impact was immediate.

In *Witness to AIDS*, Edwin Cameron's compelling memoir, he grapples with the meaning of HIV/AIDS: for himself as he confronts the possibility of his own lingering death, and for all of us in facing up to one of the most desperate challenges of our time.

In his intensely personal account of survival, Cameron blends elements of his destitute childhood with his daily duties as a senior judge and international human rights lawyer, while focusing always on the epidemic's central issues: stigma, unjust discrimination, and, most vitally, the life-and-death question of access to treatment.

Cameron's remarkable story of his own survival in an epidemic that has cost millions of lives is at once moving and uplifting, sobering and ultimately hopeful.

Edwin Cameron is a Justice in the Supreme Court of Appeal, South Africa and an internationally respected human rights lawyer and AIDS campaigner. He is an Honorary Fellow of Keble College, Oxford, and of the Society for Advanced Legal Studies, London. He also holds a Special Award from the Bar of England and Wales for his contribution to international jurisprudence and the protection of human rights. He has been awarded the San Francisco AIDS Foundation Excellence in Leadership Award.

Witness to AIDS

Edwin Cameron

With contributions by Nathan Geffen

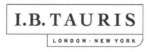
I.B. TAURIS
LONDON · NEW YORK

Published in 2005 by I.B.Tauris & Co Ltd
6 Salem Road, London W2 4BU
175 Fifth Avenue, New York NY 10010
www.ibtauris.com

In the United States of America and in Canada distributed by
Palgrave Macmillan, a division of St Martin's Press
175 Fifth Avenue, New York NY 10010

First published in South Africa by Tafelberg Publishers Limited

ISBN 1 84511 119 2 paperback
EAN 978 1 84511 119 9 paperback

A full CIP record for this book is available from the British Library
A full CIP record for this book is available from the Library of
Congress

Library of Congress catalog card: available

Typeset in ITC Veljovic
Printed and bound in Great Britain by MPG Books Ltd, Bodmin

'For these survivors, remembering is a duty. They do not want to forget, and above all they do not want the world to forget, because they understand that their experiences were not meaningless...'

For the Richters –
Jeanie, Wim, Marlise and Graham

Contents

Foreword
By Nelson Mandela

Edwin Cameron is an important South African who has made lasting contributions in many fields, not least the law. I am delighted that he is now adding to his titles that of 'author', and I have no doubt that this book will contribute to the greater good in the same way that he has done in other areas of life.

It is as a campaigner in the HIV/AIDS pandemic that Edwin has been most readily recognisable as a public figure in recent years and, as someone living with AIDS himself, his witness and activism have shown the hallmarks of great bravery and principle that I have long associated with his name.

Several years ago, I sent a message in support of Edwin, who was to deliver the Diana, Princess of Wales Lecture on AIDS. I said it was a particular privilege to pay tribute to him as one of South Africa's new heroes: as a human rights lawyer and now Justice in our country, his record is a testimony to his convictions and integrity. I added that as an AIDS activist he had demonstrated a level of courage and humanity that inspired many people into action. I reiterate that message now, and hope that the publication of his story will mean that still more people come to understand that this pandemic demands action in the same way that the struggle against apartheid demanded action.

I hope that every person who reads this book will feel encouraged to make a contribution to the campaign to provide the means and resources to end the pandemic. AIDS and the stigma attached to it remains one of the greatest challenges for all of us wherever we live, and it is voices like Edwin's that will remind us, and keep on reminding us, that no one should sleep easily until the disease is defeated.

Edwin Cameron was courageous in publicly declaring his status.

He is an example to all that one can live with that status and continue to make a meaningful contribution to achieving a better life for all. This book will, I am certain, be a further major contribution by this courageous South African towards that quest for a better life for all.

NR MANDELA
February 2005

1 | Second chances

I knew that I had AIDS when I could no longer climb the stairs from the judges' common room in the High Court to my chambers two floors above. For nearly three years, every morning after tea, I made a point of walking. Two flights, four landings, forty stairs. But on that day in late October 1997 I couldn't. Each step seemed an insuperable effort. My energy seemed to have drained from my legs. I was perspiring grey exhaustion. My lungs felt waterlogged. My mouth rough and dry. No pain. Just overwhelming weariness.

And fear.

After twenty steps I paused on the midway landing to lean my forehead against the wall. The stairwell was quiet. I could hear myself panting. I grimaced. The thought – that thought – could no longer be postponed. I would have to see my doctor. This afternoon.

But already I knew what he would say. It was what somehow I had been waiting for – fearing, dreading, denying, as it encircled me, closing in, for twelve years. My mouth and lungs told me what I didn't want to know, didn't need to be told. I had AIDS.

Acquired immunodeficiency syndrome. An accumulation of rare afflictions of the human body. Uncommon lung infections. Unusual cancers. Disabling funguses. Running unbridled through the body – because the immune system no longer functions. Threatening debilitation and portending a lingering death.

I already knew a lot about AIDS. That it is caused by HIV – a rare kind of virus that destroys a type of white blood cell in the human body, the helper T or CD4 + T cells. These are vital to the body's defences against disease. HIV targets them. Because it cannot replicate on its own, the virus enters the helper T cells – the very cells that produce the body's defence mechanisms against disease – and cannibalises the cell mechanisms to reproduce itself. As HIV destroys more and more CD4 cells, the immune system becomes weaker, less able to ward off new infections. Each illness in turn weakens the body further and renders it less able to fight HIV – causing a terrible cycle of wasting illnesses that culminate in death.

All this I knew. In fact, I knew too much. I didn't want to know more. Specifically I didn't want to know that HIV had finally succeeded in getting the better of my own immune system. That I had reached the diagnostic point where I was not 'just' living with HIV (a last consoling defence) – but that I actually had AIDS. And that without immediate, expert intervention I faced near-certain death.

In that southern spring of 1997 there was much in my life that was good, that I wanted to build on. Apart from deeply supportive family relationships (and a new love affair, later to prove misguided), my work as a High Court judge was challenging and interesting. The Johannesburg High Court is South Africa's busiest superior court. As a former human rights lawyer – one whose practice as an advocate did not focus on commercial cases – I wanted to meet the challenge of getting on top of the intricate contractual and company law problems and insolvencies the court roll presented each day. Most of all I was determined to keep up. Every judge in Johannesburg works under remorseless pressure. I didn't want to let anyone down. But even more I didn't want to admit to myself – couldn't afford to admit to myself, still less to colleagues – that I was desperately ill.

So as increasing tiredness took hold of me, as my body stopped digesting food and I lost appetite and weight, as I felt more and more shortness of breath, my response was to stretch my working hours, to cut out alcohol and late evenings to conserve energy, to bury myself in books and files so that I could stay abreast. To stop work would be to admit defeat. And admitting defeat meant death.

That week the judge-president (the senior judge in the division, who allocates the work) nominated me to a two-judge panel whose purpose was to decide appeals from the magistrates' decisions. Our caseload involved appeals against convictions and sentences in criminal cases (drugs, rapes, assault, robbery, murder) as well as civil appeals (car crashes, contractual clashes, disputes between landlords and tenants). The long and demanding case lists required advance preparation over weekends and in the evenings. The senior colleague sitting with me was a wine connoisseur, a refined and courteous man who treated both agreement and disagreement with cordiality.

The previous day one of our cases had already brought disagreement. For some reason this collegial difference triggered an especial attentiveness in me. A young man had submitted a false insurance claim for a stolen car and its contents. This made him guilty of the criminal offence of fraud. When he was arrested, the insurance company was busy processing his claim for his Opel Kadett. A second claim for the belongings he claimed he had left inside it – compact disc player, speaker and discs, golf clubs, gym kit and sunglasses – had already been paid out to him in insurance benefits. His conduct undoubtedly constituted a serious misdemeanour.

A prisons' social worker recommended a soft option – instead of jail the young man should be house-arrested and made to undergo counselling and perform community service. In favour of this was his clean record. On being caught out he owned up and pleaded guilty. He didn't waste the court's time. And, importantly, since his crime he had managed to get another job and was repaying the insurance company what it had paid out to him. At his trial he offered a belated apology.

The magistrate disregarded the prison worker's recommendation. He sentenced the young man to twelve months' jail. Was this justifiable? For us as judges hearing the appeal, it was a borderline case. We could intervene only if the sentencing magistrate's reasons contained an error, or if the sentence imposed was shockingly heavy. As it happened, the magistrate had gone wrong in some of his reasoning. So technically we were entitled to intervene, and impose a new sentence. But the real question was not technical: it was – jail or community service? My colleague and I both hesitated. Before hearing the appeal, we talked it through carefully. He tended to think we should confirm the magistrate's sentence. This sort of fraud was serious. And insurance scams were mounting, costing honest consumers hundreds of millions in extra premiums. The courts needed to send a clear message to middle-class offenders – those who used paper, and the opportunities their relative affluence in a poor society offered them, to commit crime. Jail was not only for street thieves and housebreakers and robbers. 'White collar' crimes could and sometimes rightly should also land you in jail.

Despite this, my own initial inclination was that the jail sentence was unjustifiably harsh. Both of us were open to persuasion, and each felt that he could persuade the other. During argument the young man's advocate urged us to set aside the jail sentence. His opponent from the state prosecution office defended it. After the arguments my sense that we should use our appellate powers to intervene clarified and firmed within me. I thought that the young man should get a crucial second chance. That evening I worked late to type up a draft judgment setting out the reasons why. Sitting at my laptop in my study at home I could hear my own breathing. My chest felt heavy, my breath short. But I had to finish the draft. Later, I fell into a damp, unrefreshing sleep. In the morning I handed my draft reasons to my colleague. When I saw him at tea just before my standstill in the stairwell, he promised to think it through.

Thoughts about this case, and others, were close to my mind. But as I leaned against the landing wall they threatened to recede beyond reach. I did not want to be falling ill. Not think myself ill. Not face death. Not face telling my colleagues – or having colleagues suspect, conclude – that I had AIDS.

My doctor's receptionist fitted me in immediately after court that day. While I sat in the waiting room she brought me a mug of tea. Though it had cooled by the time I took it into the consultation room, I winced painfully as I took the first sip. My doctor picked this up immediately. He looked concerned. 'That's a sure sign of thrush right through your oesophagus, Edwin,' he said. 'It's what's making it so difficult for you to swallow. And it's also why you've lost so much weight. Apart from what the virus is doing to your body, your system just can't absorb food any more,' he explained.

I smiled grimly at my doctor. David Johnson is a spry man who wears crisply ironed shirts and serves his practice and his patients with energetic determination. I had been in his care for six years, and had come to depend on his sympathetic professionalism. Over the previous months he had been tracking my CD4 and viral load counts with increasing regularity to measure my immune system and the virus's rampaging progress. It was already clear to both of us that my immune system was declining. But it was a stop-start process. For a long time my immune system had been mostly heading downwards. But occasionally it would show an upward spurt. Until that afternoon it had not seemed irreversibly clear that I would fall ill with AIDS or when I would. And once I did, the most difficult question confronted us: what to do about it?

The year before, in July 1996, New York City AIDS clinician Dr David Ho made a dramatic announcement at a conference in Vancouver. Trials across North America had shown what was previously unthinkable – that the virus could be stopped in its tracks. The first AIDS case was formally diagnosed in June 1981. For more than a decade and a half, repeated hopes that modern medicine could beat the disease proved false. Those infected with HIV, with virtually no exceptions, went on to develop AIDS. And almost everyone who developed AIDS died. It was a simple, grim, inevitable prognosis.

That inevitability medical science now seemed to have overcome. For the first time, it seemed that doctors could deal with the disease – by administering a closely monitored package of antiretroviral drugs. Previous attempts to treat AIDS with one or even two antiretrovirals had failed. The virus soon found a way around them, emerging stronger and more resilient. But new types of anti-HIV drugs were constantly being developed – particularly a new class that stopped HIV from breaking up the proteins it needs to produce new viral particles. And Ho and his colleagues now realised that using more drugs of different types in combination with each other was the key. Triple (or in some cases quadruple) therapy, with drugs chosen for their different angles of attack on the virus's means of replicating, were now proving dramatically successful in keeping it at bay. 'Highly active antiretroviral therapy' (HAART) was medicine's best answer yet to AIDS – and it looked extremely promising. Doctors were talking about 'long-term viral suppression'. And if patients kept taking the right drugs in the right combinations, it looked as though it might even be permanent.

At first some doctors went so far as to hope that over time the new drugs would eliminate the virus from the body completely by stopping viral replication. That would go beyond treatment. It would be a cure. But such hopes proved to be over-optimistic. In the face of the drug onslaught, the virus craftily recedes into the nooks and crannies of the body (the lymph nodes, the testes, the brain membrane), into 'viral reservoirs', where current forms of treatment cannot reach it. When the patient stops taking the drug combinations, the virus in most cases emerges, rampant once more.

Even so, talk of long-term viral suppression was an astounding breakthrough. For the first time in the fifteen-year struggle with AIDS, medical science offered patients the hope of escaping what had previously been certain suffering and eventual death. After Ho's experimental results were released, other doctors adopted his breakthrough methods. For nearly a year and a half, doctors had been administering different antiretroviral drug combinations to tens of thousands of sick and dying patients throughout North America and Western Europe.

The results were astounding. In the rich world, deaths from AIDS plummeted downwards. AIDS illnesses – those that were bringing my own life to a standstill – had almost been eliminated. Once treatment stopped the virus from replicating, ravaged immune systems recovered. And the body, once more healthy, could fight off opportunistic infections.

'Lazarus' stories from the wealthy world reached us in South Africa – dramatic, first-hand accounts of patients in the very last stages of their battle with AIDS, who were saved from their deathbeds and restored to life. In the bright December sunshine of Perth, Western Australia, where I addressed a conference on HIV at the end of 1999, Graham Lovelock, one of the organisers, told me his story. At the end of November 1995 he had been admitted to hospital with dwindling health and a poor prognosis. He seemed beyond hope. Every drug had been tried and his body was at the limit of its fight against the virus's effects. His family and friends had virtually resigned themselves to his imminent death; he did not himself expect to leave hospital again. But a doctor at the hospital managed to get him onto an early trial of the new drugs. In due course he arose from his bed, not dead, but very much alive and more or less restored to health.

The stories from Sydney, Los Angeles, New York, London and Munich were the same. Flushed with excitement, *Time* magazine made Dr David Ho its 'man of the year' for 1996. The end of the first phase of the struggle with AIDS had been reached: there was a way to manage it medically over the long term.

But the good news had a dismal side to it. In 1997 the drugs were unimaginably expensive. Drug companies protected their intellectual property rights – their right to stop competing companies and poor nations from using the knowledge needed to produce and distribute the drugs – with ferocious zeal. Their commercial interests – and, they claimed, their ability to carry out further expensive life-saving research – depended on the huge profits that patent exclusivity brought them. And Western governments, particularly the United States, supported them. While patent exclusivity lasted, the companies charged as much as they could for the drugs.

In wealthy countries, the public health services were simply buying the drugs for AIDS patients at the astronomical prices. But in Africa – where the huge majority of the world's people with AIDS and HIV live – prices were a death-delivering obstacle. Only the miniscule number of people with AIDS who could afford to pay the cost of combination therapy from their own pockets stood to benefit from the new treatment. The breakthrough was perfected just as the epidemic was starting to show its most catastrophic effects in central and southern Africa. Yet the benefits of treatment were denied to those most desperately in need.

In this setting my own position was one of exceptional privilege. My job as a High Court judge paid well. At the end of 1997 my High Court job was paying me pre-tax just less than R30 000 per month [the equivalent of roughly US$4 000]. This was much less than leading lawyers earned in private practice. But it was about eight times the average salary of employees in the business sector – and almost thirty times the average monthly income of all South Africans taken together. This put me in an income bracket beyond the dreams of most of Africa's 700 million people – and also of most of the continent's thirty million people living with AIDS and HIV.

So I had choices – the choices that relative affluence conferred. The question was how to exercise them. Apart from my visits to Dr

Johnson I was – with his conditional support – seeing a homoeopath. Sensibly, although disavowing the primacy of conventional Western medicine, she recognised that homoeopathic treatment could have limits. She made few promises. 'I can keep you free from infections. And I will certainly try to keep your immune system as healthy as possible. But if the virus becomes too strong for my remedies, you will have to turn back to conventional medical treatment.' For ordinary infections, she gave me remedies free from antibiotics that not only seemed to heal but also comforted. In the six years I'd been seeing her, I felt I had benefited.

But my panting breath and my clogged throat showed that homoeopathy had not managed to stop the virus from running rampant through my body. So the big decision was whether I should start with antiretroviral drug treatment. I was what AIDS specialists called 'treatment-naive'. My body had never been exposed to any AIDS drugs, and seldom to any antibiotics – I was an ideal candidate for successful treatment.

At my last meeting with Dr Johnson, in September, my CD4 count had for the first time dipped below 200 – a clear sign of imminent AIDS. (The CD4 count of a normally healthy person is well over 800.) At this time Dr Johnson warned me: 'If you want to carry on seeing how long you can manage without starting on the antiretroviral drugs, that's fine. But as your doctor my formal advice to you has to be that you should start medication now.' He treated me as a well-informed patient with the ability to make my own choices – and wanted me to have maximum freedom. So he gave me all the facts I could possibly need to make an informed choice. (Sometimes he gave me too many. He had the alertness of a puppy, and its eagerness. Sometimes I couldn't deal with it. I wanted him to stop showing me how up-to-date he was. 'I am not here as a judge or lawyer or policy-maker. I am a patient! I want solace and guidance – not expositions of virological learning or the latest treatment breakthroughs!')

Given my doctor's on-the-record advice, why was I so reluctant to start treatment, especially when it was showing such promise? One reason was the side effects I knew that I could expect. The drugs are immensely powerful. They have to be. Powerful enough to reach into the abstruse corners of the body's genetic mechanisms, where HIV replicates, to put a stop to its machinations. So powerful that in doing so they unavoidably affect other body functions – upsetting the digestive system, causing painful nerve abreactions (tingling, numbness) and redistribution of body fat. Rare toxic reactions, some even fatal – when patients or their damaged livers just cannot tolerate the force of the drugs – gave me additional pause.

I also feared something starker: that the drugs wouldn't work for me. Dr Johnson told me that his colleagues in rich countries were reporting success rates of about 70 per cent. Wonderful. But this also meant that for almost one-third of those starting on treatment in 1997 the drugs did not work. What if I was amongst them? Reported success rates on antiretroviral therapies are now well over 90 per cent – partly because many of the first patients who started on combination therapy in the mid-1990s had in desperation tried each of the drugs one by one, making the adaptive virus wary and resilient to any further onslaught. In Africa that problem barely existed. But in 1997 doctors didn't fully appreciate the importance of 'drug naivety'. So the thought of treatment failure chilled me, dragging me from exhausted sleep at four in the morning to blinking wakefulness in the dark. What if this was it?

To postpone starting on the drugs delayed constructive action. But it seemed to keep hope alive. And, until now, apart from increasing tiredness, I wasn't actually showing any symptoms. I relied on the grinding treadmill of work in the Johannesburg High Court as an ally. As I grew more tired, I worked harder to try to keep up. And that, I reasoned, was why I was getting more tired. The self-deception was neat (denial comes in many forms). As long as it wasn't AIDS.

But on the stairwell on Tuesday morning 21 October 1997 this reasoning fell apart. I was critically short of breath. And even though I had stayed up late working on my draft judgment the night before, this, I knew, was not from overwork. Dr Johnson asked me to take my shirt off. I sat with my legs dangling uncomfortably over the edge of his high examination table. Carefully pressing his stethoscope to the front and back of my chest, he listened to my breathing. 'You don't need to listen,' I tried to keep it light. 'I can tell you that it's PCP.' In Africa the main killer of AIDS patients is tuberculosis. In the 1980s, among the gay men of North America, it was PCP – pneumocystis carinii pneumonia. An ordinary fungus, commonly found in the lungs of humans and mammals, causes it. Most toddlers in most families have been exposed to pneumocystis. To healthy adults it can do no harm, lurking in the lungs without causing any noticeable trouble.

But to malnourished youngsters – and to adults suffering from immune debilitation – it can be fatal. The latent, harmless infection flares up into a rare type of pneumonia that before AIDS was virtually unknown. Unless treated, the pneumonia is lethal. The website of the United States Centers for Disease Control (CDC) still intones with simple bluntness that in such cases 'increasing pulmonary involvement leads to death'.

But PCP is difficult to diagnose – especially in an otherwise healthy, strong adult. Although my body's increasingly unsuccessful struggle with the virus had wasted away 10 kg, I still had 85 kg left – leaving even my tall, 193 cm (nearly 6 foot 4 inches), frame hardly skeletal. Certainly I was thin – 'overworked' of course – but I by no means seemed AIDS-wasted. No one seemed to think I had AIDS. Only the previous week in a lift crowded with judges on their way to court a colleague, burly herself, had commented how thin I was. 'Are you dieting?' she challenged as I stuttered. She would have been appalled to know the truth. Just as appalled as I felt as Dr Johnson rubbed his stethoscope bup-bup-bup over my chest. He looked worried but uncertain. 'It seems like PCP, Edwin,' he said. 'But we'd better send you for X-rays.'

After court the next afternoon I found myself in the waiting room of a radiology practice in one of Johannesburg's smart private clinics. I'd spoken to no one about my incipient diagnosis. As the registrar called the cases and my colleague and I disposed of appeal after appeal, I tried to still my panic every time the thought came up. My life seemed to be fracturing in two. In one, I was a working part of the justice administration in newly democratic South Africa – an extraordinary privilege for anyone – even more so for a white person privileged by apartheid, who had thought that democracy would never happen. Judges faced enormous challenges. A fearsome crime wave was beginning to make the public, black and white, sceptical about the principles underlying our ambitious constitution. Were the new rights benefiting only criminals? Despite the clamour, President Mandela's government, and that of his successor President Mbeki, remained true to their commitment to constitutionalism. Judges and the constitution were at the centre of this debate. It was hard not to feel some significance in our work – and a sense of promise. I wanted desperately to continue, not to be sick.

But the other part of my life was washing away beneath my feet, eroded by microbes and attacked by fungi coursing through my veins and wasting my muscles and bodily reserves, leaving me tired and panicked and isolated in the waiting room. The radiologist's assistant called me in. I stripped off my jacket and shirt and donned a flimsy examination gown for her to take the X-rays. Her brisk efficiency as she manipulated the heavy X-ray negatives made me feel even more isolated. 'Dr Jacobs will see you in about twenty minutes to discuss his assessment,' she promised.

But twenty minutes passed, and then thirty. Once more in my suit, I waited in the corridor outside the viewing room. I had never been more conscious of my breathing. As the doctors walked in and out, one in particular glanced several times at me. But still I was not called in. Eventually my mobile phone rang. It was Dave Johnson. 'The radiologist has just phoned. He's sitting with your X-rays. But he can't believe what they tell him. He's scared of giving you a wrong diagnosis. He says they seem to show PCP. But he can't believe it. He says you don't look like you have AIDS. So he phoned me first to check whether you are at risk.' Dr Johnson suggested that I bring the X-rays to his home that night to double-check.

I felt helplessness mixed with despair. If the radiologist was thinking media stereotypes, of course I didn't 'look' like someone with AIDS. I was not in bed. I was not emaciated or entubed. I was fresh from a long working day in court – still in a suit. My medical insurance details at reception must have revealed my judicial status. And judges don't get AIDS. (Nor are they gay.) In any event, Dr Jacobs' practice didn't look as though many black or gay patients – those most 'at risk' – frequented it.

At last he called me in. He spread out the X-rays on his light table. Both lungs shone bright with the telltale signs of PCP. He pointed out its white spots crowding both organs. His manner was kindly, respectful. My doctor would prescribe highly effective antibiotics, he reassured me. This usually cleared the infection within ten or fourteen days. I should come back then for a further check.

That evening I took the X-rays to Dave Johnson's home. He held them up to his study lamp. 'Yes, that's what I thought, Edwin,' he said. I had AIDS. On the way home I stopped at the pharmacy to pick up the fourteen-day course of bactrim he had prescribed. And faced a long, hard evening alone at home.

People sometimes say that they couldn't go on living if they knew that they had HIV. Or that they'd 'just' kill themselves if they ever got AIDS. It's a stupid and unreflective thought. I know, because I used to think it myself. I used to tell myself that I could not carry on living if I were ever diagnosed with full-blown AIDS. Then, I fancied, life could surely not be worth continuing. So I would take the simple course. I would just allow PCP – or whatever horrific opportunistic infection arrived to herald AIDS – to take its course, and let my too too solid flesh melt, thaw and resolve itself into a dew. Without treatment PCP would make quick despatch of me.

Reality is less poetic. Or it was for me. Impending death did not arrive gracefully in the form of sensible choices. It was fetid, frightening, intrusive, oppressive. Too often I had seen friends and comrades die of AIDS. Had seen how day by day, week by week, they would redefine wellness, adjusting it downwards each time, but never losing its goal, no matter how wasted, disabled or physically dysfunctional they became. Getting better always seems to remain attainable, even when from the outside it was plain that it no longer was. I had seen too many friends choose life, right until the end, even when they knew – must have known? – that it was receding from them, no longer an option, that it was death only that awaited them.

Like them, I now experienced no existential hesitation. I just wanted to keep on living. I wanted my health back. Urgently. I wanted to breathe easily, freely again. I could not let diagnoses of PCP and all that they seemed to imply get in the way. And I had plenty to distract me. My imprudently chosen lover seemed to want to play a game of chase. Perhaps my inner commotion was more palpable to those closest to me than I had thought. To them I spoke about HIV.

And to some I even mentioned PCP – or just 'a chest infection'. But the accompanying diagnosis and its implications I did not reveal. The word AIDS was too big, too frightening, too fraught with implication. Too final.

My sister Jeanie, who for forty years had nurtured and protected me, worried over the phone. She listened carefully to what I described of my visits to Dave and the radiologist, and urged me to get into bed. I refused. How could I? There was court work to be done. The judge-president had included me on the roster of duties for the rest of the year. And I had meetings to attend. And committees to run. I was needed. Thank goodness. When Jeanie offered to travel the 60 km from Pretoria to Johannesburg to bring me meals, I assured her that it wasn't necessary.

To accept sympathy and support means acknowledging weakness and dependency. I wasn't ready for this. AIDS had to wait. Months before, Judge-President Eloff had circulated a court roll posting me to a six-week out-of-town session of the High Court. The circuit was due to begin on Monday in Vereeniging, an industrial riverside town ninety minutes' drive from Johannesburg. I had already arranged for two young lawyers – promising black practitioners at the Johannesburg Bar – to join me on the bench as assessors. For them the work would bring good exposure. For me (like most white South Africans, miserably only bilingual in a country where people generally speak four or more languages) their assistance in understanding issues and clarifying meaning would be indispensable. While I would determine legal questions alone, on factual issues we would vote together – and in case of disagreement their vote could prevail. Both had set aside time – and perhaps turned away briefs – to perform this public service on the Bench with me. So cancelling the Vereeniging circuit seemed unthinkable . . . Of course it was. Apart from anything, getting into bed and acknowledging how sick I was would cause talk. And that was unthinkable . . .

On the Monday we started the daily drive to the Vereeniging circuit court. I was relieved to have an agreeable young clerk do the driving while I leaned back into the passenger seat, willing the antibiotics to work as quickly as possible. Some of the cases on our roll came from Sharpeville, a township adjoining Vereeniging with intense historical associations. Twice in thirty years the name focused world attention on the excesses of apartheid – first when white police killed some sixty unarmed protesters at the Sharpeville police station in March 1960; and a second time twenty-five years later when a judge sentenced six township activists to death in December 1985 for the murder of a local councillor serving in apartheid structures.

When the first Sharpeville disaster happened I was five weeks from my seventh birthday – newly arrived with my older sisters Laura and Jean at a children's home in Queenstown in the Eastern Cape province. Some of the other children were orphans, others had been abandoned. Most were from impoverished broken homes, their parents unable to care for them. My older siblings and I fell into the last category. After a succession of moves from city to town and back to city, as my alcoholic father drank his way out of job after job, our fragmented family finally fell apart. My mother, sad and angry and not coping at all, finally gave up on the marriage and divorced him a second time. Well-meaning church friends persuaded her that it was best to send us 700 km away to the children's home.

If news of the Sharpeville massacre reached us there – and it surely did, for the Eastern Cape was alive with resistance to apartheid rule – it had to contend with other issues to make a mark on my boyish perceptions. There was talk of attacks by 'Poqo', the 'pure' armed resistance wing of the Pan Africanist Congress, a breakaway faction from the African National Congress. We were told that attacks were imminent. I imagined black warriors like those depicted in the stilted history books the older children used, streaming over the hilltops surrounding Queenstown.

The intervening twenty-five years transformed not only my circumstances but my consciousness. Queenstown seemed very far away. But the journey from the children's home had left me with an intense, central, motivating awareness. There were many poor, deprived children in South Africa. Many intelligent, ambitious children, willing to work and to strive. Many who yearned for escape, release, transcendence from constricting material circumstance and poverty. What made me different from most of them was my skin colour. What made me different was that the country was structured to privilege me while systematically disadvantaging others. What saved me from poverty was that I was white. After nearly five years in the children's home, and a series of further schools in various parts of the country, my mother, despite her own poverty, managed at last to secure me a place in a first-rate government high school for boys. Set on a hill overlooking Pretoria's most affluent suburbs, Sir Herbert Baker's early twentieth century buildings were designed to epitomise the grace and dignity and scholarship appropriate to questing male adolescence. Arriving on the first day shortly before my fourteenth birthday, I felt nearly suffocated with apprehension and excitement. I craved all the elegant learning Pretoria Boys' High School seemed to offer, and all the opportunities beyond that. I could hardly believe that all this had become available to me.

The school changed my life. What I learned there – perhaps even more importantly, those I met there – gave me access to rich opportunities. These included the fulsome Anglo American Corporation open scholarship that enabled me to study law and English and Latin and Greek at Stellenbosch (a lovely university town near Cape Town whose oak-lined streets are filled with Cape-Dutch architecture), and later one of the world's very best openings – three years at Oxford as a Rhodes Scholar. Back from Oxford, I joined the Johannesburg Bar as an advocate. But in the growing crisis of apartheid a commercial practice did not attract or satisfy me. It seemed imperative that if law should survive as a way of regulating social conflict in South Africa – if it deserved to survive at all – more lawyers should get involved in fighting injustice in the courts and by offering legal advice and support to organisations and individuals resisting apartheid. Through November 1985, as I packed up my fledgling commercial practice to move to full-time work as a public interest lawyer at the University of the Witwatersrand's Centre for Applied Legal Studies, I closely followed reports about a murder trial that, twenty-five years after the original Sharpeville tragedy, was once again bringing that name into resonant public prominence throughout the world.

The gruesome murder on 3 September 1984 of Jacob Kuzwayo Dlamini, an apartheid-structure councillor, by an enraged crowd of township residents, produced a grim atmosphere when eight Sharpeville residents were put on trial for their lives in 1985. Defence advocates told of a hostile judge and a determined prosecutor. Even so, when six death sentences were pronounced in December 1985 (two of the accused were acquitted), they came as a shock. For my own part, I knew that, beyond any question of individual moral accountability, the underlying iniquities of apartheid were to blame for the growing cycle of violence that was sweeping the country. As a white South African, I saw that the executions would only add to the injustice and resistant rage that apartheid had spawned. And as a human rights lawyer, the way in which the courts I operated in daily dealt with the case left me appalled and angry.

The trial judge sentenced all six to the gallows, even though the prosecution could not prove that the actions of each had actually contributed to Dlamini's death. The case of one of the condemned six shocked me particularly. Fearing for his life, the embattled councillor had fired a shot that wounded one of a hundred-strong crowd surrounding his house. In response, a young woman named Theresa Ramashamola was found to have shouted: 'He's shooting at us, let us kill him.' Others certainly heard her. But in the hubbub, who could say that her cries had actually heightened tensions, incited the perpetrators, hastened the murder? The court heard no such evidence. Later, when someone pleaded that the injured councillor should not be burned, Theresa slapped her. For these words she was not only convicted of murder but the judge refused to find 'extenuating circumstances', which would have permitted a jail sentence. He sentenced her to hang. I was aghast.

The case of another accused appalled me as much. None of the witnesses placed him on the scene of the crime. Unlike the other accused, he was arrested more than two months after the murder. One of those directly linked to the murder took the police to his home to retrieve the dead man's firearm that the killers had wrested from him in his dying moments. When confronted by the police, the accused man readily produced the weapon from a hiding place in his ceiling. He had taken it, he claimed, from youths who were nearby on the day of the murder. He denied being present at the murder.

The judge disbelieved his evidence – he had lied about events at his house; he couldn't explain why the other accused knew that the firearm was with him; and in court he falsely disputed that the weapon produced in court was identical to the one he had retrieved from his ceiling for the police.

Was this enough to hang a man? Was this enough to conclude beyond reasonable doubt that he was the very man who had wrested the deceased's firearm from him in his death struggle? Did his lies together with possession of the crucial weapon prove that he was one of the killers? Surely not. The firearm was retrieved from him nine weeks after the murder. English judges had developed a logical way to link someone caught red-handed with an incriminating object to a recently committed crime. South African judges adopted it – the 'doctrine of recent possession'. But it had never been applied after so long a delay. No civilised system, I thought, could do so. After nine weeks the possessor of the incriminating firearm could not possibly be described as 'red-handed'. And however many lies he told, there was a substantial – and, I thought, obvious – chance that he had come into possession of the dead man's weapon in a way that did not implicate him in the murder.

Well, why then did he lie? South African courts treat a lying accused with scant sympathy. But a number of authoritative judgments warned that a criminal defendant might lie for reasons other than that he was guilty. In the case of this accused, it seemed more than reasonable – indeed, I thought, obvious – to assume that he might have lied about when and how he got the firearm because he didn't want to implicate the co-accused who had brought the police to him. To exculpate himself, he would have had to say, 'I took the weapon from him and agreed to hide it in my ceiling because he told me he got it from the dead man at the time of his murder.' Was it unreasonable to suppose that the motive for his trivial lies was a reluctance to 'snitch' on his friend – particularly given the fraught racial and political tensions surrounding Dlamini's murder and the police investigation?

To me the verdict seemed an outrageous curvature of the laws of logic and fairness – a miscarriage of justice symptomatic of the extremities apartheid was inflicting on the legal system.

But the trial judge decided otherwise. And five judges of appeal in the appeal court in Bloemfontein confirmed his verdict. Incensed, I became vocal in an international campaign to save 'the Sharpeville

Six'. I wrote an article for a scholarly journal. I addressed meetings. I spoke to foreign correspondents posted to Johannesburg. Three weeks before the six were due to stand on the gallows, after the government had refused to commute their sentences, I attacked the verdicts in an opinion piece in the mass-circulation Johannesburg *Sunday Times*. I pointed a finger at the appeal court for 'widening the doctrines of criminal liability in response to evidence of township revolt'. My criticisms were quoted in London newspapers, where a distinguished former law lord, Lord Scarman, and a senior British barrister who observed the trial, Louis Blom-Cooper QC, also attacked the outcome. When one of the prosecution witnesses recanted his evidence, the unflagging lawyer for the six, Prakash Diar, asked me to join the team fighting for their lives by applying to re-open the case.

But those defending the courts' verdict counterattacked. Chief Justice Rabie was greatly offended. He sent a message through Judge-President Moll to the Johannesburg Bar Council, asking the body to institute disciplinary steps against me. To its credit, the Council voted overwhelmingly (though not unanimously) against any sanction.

The year before, the minister of justice in State President PW Botha's cabinet, Kobie Coetsee, had attacked me for accusing three prominent judges of pro-apartheid collusion. His official statement slated me, 'the young Mr Cameron,' as a 'lesser known officer of the court'. He dismissed my criticism of the judiciary as 'distasteful and improper'. He added for good measure that I appeared to derive 'some sort of misguided pleasure from denigrating great Chief Justices'. Now at a national Bar conference Chief Justice Rabie himself condemned my criticism of the verdict, saying it was little short of 'shocking and disgraceful'. In a later case the appeal judge who authored the Sharpeville Six judgment took the unprecedented step of responding to the criticism, saying that he had ignored 'the misguided comments of hysterical politicians masquerading as lawyers'. It was a bad jibe. But what it showed was that criticism of the verdict had certainly found its mark.

I refused to apologise. There seemed to be nothing to apologise for. My criticism to me seemed well justified – even mild. It stood out only because during the 1980s few lawyers in practice or at universities within South Africa dared to criticise apartheid judges. At Wits

University, two gifted colleagues, Etienne Mureinik (who later died tragically by his own hand) and Carole Lewis, wrote to the press defending my right to criticise. And they organised a colloquium to discuss my intervention. But from other legal and academic institutions there was mainly a deathly reverential hush. Books critical of the South African legal system, by lawyers associated with the exiled African National Congress, were prohibited from circulation. In this near vacuum, outspoken challenges resounded loudly.

Instead of backing down from my public criticism, I threw myself into the court bid to reopen the case of the Six. The recanting prosecution witness had earned them a merciful reprieve. The afternoon before they were due to hang the trial judge, in a lifesaving fit of doubt – aware no doubt of the international outrage – granted them a temporary reprieve to plead for a new trial. Shortly afterwards I visited them on death row. In the corner of the cramped warder's office where we met there was a scale. Next to it stood a vertically adjustable wooden device with centimetre markings. They told me that the day before their scheduled execution the hangman had carefully weighed and measured them. He had to calculate exactly what length of rope was necessary to kill each of them efficiently.

In the 1980s, South Africa had one of the highest number of recorded hangings in the world. In 1987, no fewer than 164 people were hanged. One almost every second day. Executions were carried out in a severely guarded, bleak new cell block in Pretoria's maximum security prison. I visited death row only three or four times. Each time I left chilled within. To reach it one had to cross a final quadrangle with painstakingly nurtured lawns and flowerbeds. Inside, the windows were vertical slits, the interior drably painted, the atmosphere one of controlled desperation. In the courtyard outside, the warders kept ducks. Perhaps their necks were never wrung.

While the Six remained in their cells on death row, Sydney Kentridge, the famed South African advocate then gaining prominence at the London Bar, flew back to present the argument. We lost. But Chief Justice Rabie and his appeal court colleagues gave us a respectful hearing. And as so often under apartheid, a legal challenge, even when it did not attract a favourable judgment, helped to secure a favourable outcome. The court bid bought the six vital time. The

Sharpeville Six, too, would have a second chance. Even though the legal challenge had failed, the apartheid government could no longer afford to hang them. The international outcry had saved their lives. It had also saved the country from the explosion that was certain to have followed their executions. It had also saved, I thought, the South African judiciary from the irremediable ignominy that the deaths of the Six would surely have earned it.

In late October 1997, travelling the busy highway through the industrial heart of South Africa to start the Vereeniging circuit, I, too, yearned for a second chance at life. I was now part of the judiciary, one of the first High Court judges President Mandela had appointed in 1994 under the new democratic constitution. I wanted to fulfil my duties. And I wanted to concede as little as I possibly could to the disease that now threatened to stifle my life. The cases on the court roll that October/November in Vereeniging presented all the problems and pains of our nascent country's transition from an unjust past to the better future to which we all – lawyers, politicians, judges, people – had committed ourselves. I wanted to be part of it.

The first case my assessors and I heard involved a vigilante killing. A family claimed that the victim had murdered their uncle. They had brought the victim to their home to confront him. When he tried to escape they beat, stoned and stabbed him to death. Then they poured petrol over his body. The district surgeon told us that the flames had reduced it to charcoal. One murder had led to an even more gruesome second. My assessors and I convicted two nephews of the first victim for murdering the second. Other family members, including a sister, we acquitted, because of weak prosecution evidence. In our judgment we emphasised that justice was, or should be, the exclusive prerogative of the courts.

But mistrust of apartheid law and order had set off a grim cycle of vigilantism in many townships. Even a newly accountable police force could not perform miracles. Still too few people trusted police or courts to deal effectively with offenders. And still too few police themselves engendered that trust – as one of our next cases harrowingly showed. A packed courtroom rose as we entered to hear the prosecutor call the trial of police sergeant Jappie Masilo Twala. He faced two separate charges of murder plus two of attempted murder. When his brothers became involved in a Sunday night bar-room spat about a stolen watch, Sergeant Twala went to intervene. As tempers flared and a stone-throwing crowd gathered, he pulled out his service pistol and fired three shots. One of the shots proved fatal for a stone-thrower. When Sergeant Twala and his brothers fled the scene they left a corpse behind – that of a nineteen-year-old pupil at a local school.

Days passed. Yet the police did nothing. Sergeant Twala was not arrested. Was he immune? The dead youth's school friends seemed to fear that he was. On the eighth day of police inaction, they gathered at a special school assembly. There they resolved that they would confront Twala themselves. They abandoned their classes. They took to the streets and forced commuter buses to a halt. They boarded them en masse, and compelled the drivers to divert to Twala's home. Twala was out. So the crowd destroyed his home.

The house was modest but recently built, neatly middle class and well appointed. When the youths were done, it was no longer a home. In court we saw the photographs. The damage the youths had caused was literally devastating – they lit fires, broke doors, shattered windows, ripped fittings from the wall, overturned cupboards and fridges. What they didn't destroy they carried away with them. It was a terrible, unlicensed rebuke for a deed Twala had not been charged with, had not been tried for, nor convicted of. It was also vengeance born of police inaction.

Sergeant Twala was out investigating a crime. He received an urgent radio message summoning him home. He hastened back to find his household wrecked. School children were still running from the scene. Inspecting the damage, a senior colleague tried to console him. He assured Twala that three of the guilty youths were under arrest. Indeed, they were right outside, safely locked up in the back of his police van.

On hearing this Twala left the house. He went to the police van and unlocked its back doors. Precisely what followed was sharply disputed at the trial. What was certain was that a fusillade of shots was fired into the van. After it, Twala's service pistol magazine was empty. And one youth lay dead. Another was critically injured. A third was wounded. The shots had ripped through the chest of the dead youth, killing him instantly. The second they rendered a spinal paraplegic, with permanent partial paralysis of his ankles and feet. The third suffered wounds to his chest, thigh and arm. Fortunately he was not permanently injured. But in court he told my assessors and me about the psychological suffering he had endured.

Before us, Twala faced two murder charges – the stone-thrower he had shot in the spat with his brothers; and the schoolboy killed in the back of the police van. Twala denied any culpability. In the barroom brawl he had acted in necessary self-defence. At the police van, he claimed, the youths inside had set upon him when he opened the doors. In the ensuing struggle his firearm went off – quite unintentionally.

On the first killing my assessors and I found the prosecution witnesses honest. But their evidence was not sufficiently firm for a murder conviction. Everyone had been drinking, and accounts as to what had happened when differed. Besides, everyone agreed that a hostile crowd had gathered and that tempers were running high. Self-defence could not be rejected as untrue beyond reasonable doubt. Twala had to be acquitted.

But on the police van shootings we had no hesitation in rejecting his account. The two surviving youths gave pitifully convincing, unembroidered evidence of how Twala had opened the doors of the police van, produced his pistol and then wildly emptied the magazine. The district surgeon gave detailed evidence on the sites of the wound entry and exit points. He confirmed that the young men's account squared with the medical evidence. We found Twala guilty of the murder of the dead youth, and of the attempted murder of the two survivors. He was lucky not to have had the survivors' lives on his hands as well.

Even so, we found that he had not acted cold-bloodedly. He was in a desperate rage, overcome by the awful devastation he had gone home to witness. Mercy required that I take this into account in sentencing him – and that I purge from my mind suspicion about the earlier killing. I did so. Despite the death of the youngster, and the horrific injuries to the other two, I imposed a strongly mitigated sentence of nine years' imprisonment.

Twala was not content. His defence – like that of most policemen charged with on-duty killings – was conducted by the state legal office, which briefed experienced counsel. His case ended three years later in the Constitutional Court. A judgment in his name set a precedent about appeal procedures. But the murder findings and his nine-year sentence remained intact. With remission and parole, he is by now probably long out of jail. Sergeant Twala, too, has had a second chance.

After my session with the X-ray doctor, my clerk and assessors and I travelled to Vereeniging and back every day. Each morning I donned the bib, sash, waistband and flowing scarlet robes that English judges had imported to South Africa when the British took the Cape from the Dutch in colonial conquest in 1803. The resplendent robes gave me a full-body disguise. This was just as well. Despite the radiologist's confidence that the antibiotics would repel the AIDS pneumonia within ten to fourteen days, it proved to be surprisingly stubborn. Ten days into the circuit, I returned for my fourteen-day check. Studying the new X-rays with me, Dr Jacobs gave me the bad news. It had not cleared. I needed more antibiotics – in a stronger daily dose. Dr Johnson had underestimated the dose my still substantial body weight demanded.

Naturally, if I had got into bed and rested, the drugs would have had a better chance of slaying the microbial dragon raging within me. But bed rest had never seemed an option. In near despair, I returned to Dave Johnson for a further script. He gave me another week on a double dose of bactrim.

The next morning I travelled back to Vereeniging.

But the treatment was ghastly. The powerful antibiotics, in their as yet unavailing onslaught on the PCP, caused a red rash to flush out over my upper torso and face. My appetite, sparse as it was, seemed to vanish. My stomach tightened. Eating was becoming even more difficult. I lost more weight. After being diagnosed with HIV in 1990, my friend Zackie Achmat had experienced a lung infection. On the Sunday after I was diagnosed he came to visit me at home. My breathing was even more laboured than before. I did not feel at all well. It showed. Zackie knew all too well. We sat facing each other, rigid, each unable to speak the words of reassurance and comfort the other needed.

Worst of all was that the antibiotics had further suppressed my body's weakened antifungal defences. The result was the return of oral and oesophageal thrush. Dave Johnson had prescribed Diflucan – a fantastically expensive, but blessedly effective, antifungal drug. Its expense was later to trigger one of the most dramatic activist challenges to the pharmaceutical industry (which I describe in Chapter 6). For me, the cost of the tablets – about R120, or nearly US$20 a tablet: the approximate equivalent of the daily earnings of an employee in the business sector – was fortunately covered by the judges' medical insurance scheme. I thought that the precious and expensive Diflucan had done the trick. But no. One of my worst moments – I often think the worst – was one morning at the mirror, two weeks after diagnosis, when I noticed that my tongue once more was flecked with resurgent thrush. My heart sank. It felt like a defining moment, inviting despair. Fungal spores grow on dead bodies . . . The treatment hadn't beaten the PCP. The thrush was back. I was feeling ghastly. Was my body shutting down for death? Would the treatment fail me?

But I could not allow such thoughts to be more than momentary. I could not let them take hold. I was not yet a dead body. And I didn't want to become one. I wanted a second chance. Determinedly, perhaps desperately, I continued working. There was in fact much to do. A committee I had been leading since 1996 was advising the country's law commission, an influential national statutory law reform body, on AIDS. Already, several reports we had delivered had impressed the commission with their thoroughness and their powerful, well-balanced arguments. The commission had endorsed our findings and sent them on to Parliament, where they had found their way into beneficent legislation.

Now we were close to producing recommendations to ban pre-employment testing for HIV – a widespread practice that irrationally and unfairly barred job applicants with HIV from finding or taking up employment. I knew something about the effects of pre-employment HIV testing. In 1993 I started a university-based AIDS law project that offered legal services against AIDS discrimination. One of the reasons was the stream of calls for help I'd been receiving at Wits University's human rights centre. As the South African epidemic took hold, people came for help against high-handed, sometimes cruel behaviour by employers who were determined – completely impractically – to have nothing to do with AIDS: an 'AIDS-free' workforce, as some put it. Some callers were policemen, others were in the army, many were in business and in industrial concerns.

By and large the law commission committee – composed of business people, health specialists, lawyers and activists – agreed that both justice and good sense demanded that the practice be outlawed. Zackie joined soon after we started. He added fire as well as strategic wile to our discussions. We had to work out a compromise to place unanimously before the commission, and with it prepare watertight draft legislation for the commission to pass on to Parliament. It was not easy. One day I adjourned court early in Vereeniging to meet committee members in Pretoria. Soon after, we fitted in an extra Saturday meeting to finalise our proposals. None of this, I thought, could wait. And immersing myself in it somehow anaesthetised me against the panic that my bodily frailty was inducing in me.

Yet there was a tension, and a paradox. I was dealing with AIDS as a judge, chairing a committee, making public statements and important public recommendations. But I was also dealing with AIDS within myself. As the disease's symptoms raged through my body, the split between the two roles unsettled me more than ever before. I began to think that at some time, sooner rather than later, I would have to unite the public and the personal. I couldn't continue being a highly visible and respected AIDS policy advocate in public life while dealing secretly with the debilitating effects of the sickness in my own life. It wasn't a question of ethics. Despite holding public office as a judge, I was, I thought, entitled to keep my state of health to myself. But in simple practical terms it just seemed to divert too much energy. Secrecy is all too often a worrying and time-consuming and energy-sapping business. And it was just unnecessarily exhausting. These thoughts bore fruit just a short while later.

Meanwhile, the extra effort the committee put in at the end of 1997 proved thoroughly worthwhile. Early in 1998, the full commission approved our recommendations on prohibiting pre-employment testing for HIV. The recommendation that pre-employment testing for HIV be prohibited went to Parliament – and just months later a new statute enshrining workplace fairness banned all HIV testing of workers and job applicants unless special court authority was obtained from the labour court.

But the flecks I saw on my tongue and the unrelenting PCP at last persuaded me that I had to allow myself some time off for recovery. The next week offered a respite, as the case my assessors and I were currently trying was drawing to a close. Some of the later trials I could postpone to catch up on during the ensuing January's court vacation. With my heart in my mouth I called Judge-President Eloff to arrange time off. What questions would he ask? What would he say? Would he support me? As it turned out, he asked nothing. I told him that I had a chest infection and was not feeling well. He asked for no details. Instead, he assured me immediately that it was paramount that I should recover. There would be no problem if I rearranged the circuit to finish the delayed cases later.

Relieved, I put down the phone. For now at least, work could take second place. The last few weeks had taught me some important lessons. For the first time I could contemplate using a space in which I could feel better. For the first time I learned to risk relying on other people for help during my illness. And in every case their responses touched me and moved me and reassured me.

Under attack from the doubled dosage, the PCP was beginning to recede. As it did, Dave Johnson and I discussed when I would take my first dose of antiretroviral therapy. By now there was no question but that I had to start combination therapy. Even if we managed to deal with the PCP and thrush this time with ordinary medications, further HIV-induced weakness and illnesses, progressively increasing, were all that awaited me, like so many before, like so many others in Africa.

The experience of an incapable, inefficient chest and a fungus-clogged gullet had scared me right out of further ambivalence or uncertainty. If there was a chance that the treatment would fail me, there was twice as much chance that it would succeed. What distinguished me from other Africans dying of AIDS was that I had the means – though barely – to clutch at the near miraculous new remedy of antiretroviral treatment.

Dr Johnson and I agreed that I would take my first dose of antiretroviral therapy on the day I had arranged with the judge-president for my break from circuit court to begin. I told my family and some close friends – those whom I felt that I could trust with my HIV status. In a jovial, nearly festive, atmosphere, I took my first pills on Thursday evening 13 November. With a small group of friends sitting around a table on my porch in the warmth of the early summer's evening, to determined cheers I solemnly took six capsules of one of the new, breakthrough class of anti-HIV drugs – a powerful 'protease inhibitor' called ritonavir (marketed as 'Norvir').

The cost of the new treatment was enormous. The three drugs I was taking (as well as the protease inhibitor, I started taking an AZT-like drug called D4T, and another called 3TC) cost more than R4 000 (or roughly US$600) for one month's supply. This was fully one-third of my after-tax monthly income. Unless the prices of the drugs came down sharply, and soon, I would not be able to continue to afford to pay this amount every month. Too many others too close to me shared my monthly salary.

The medical insurance scheme for judges – the same one that covered members of the new democratic parliament – limited AIDS benefits of any kind to a derisory R800 per year. That amount would cover barely one-fifth of a single month's supply of my new life-saving drugs.

This surely was monstrously unfair. My fellow judges and Members of Parliament who had high blood pressure (and comparable ailments) enjoyed a chronic medication scheme of R10 000 per year – more than twelve times the maximum cap for AIDS. Why should AIDS be treated differently? Realising, as my CD4 count gradually fell, that I would at some stage need to rely on AIDS medications (or, at worst, on terminal treatment for AIDS), I had gone a year or two earlier to see a judicial colleague in Cape Town who had been specially appointed by the heads of court to represent the interests of judges on the scheme's governing board.

I had told my colleague that I had HIV – and that I feared that at some point I might fall ill with AIDS. Initially he seemed shocked and sympathetic. He promised me that he would have the unfair limit removed to equal that of comparable chronic conditions. If blood pressure or heart disease or diabetes were covered, indeed why not AIDS?

But perhaps the shock he felt at hearing that I had HIV overcame his sense of purpose. For nearly two years I sent him repeated reminders and pleas. He asked for information and statistics, which I produced. He said that he needed a memorandum to put before the board. I gave it to him. All this resulted in repeated promises, but no action. The AIDS treatment limit of R800 per year stayed. No doubt he had other things on his mind. Perhaps he temporised because he found AIDS a difficult issue.

But the extremities of illness lent me boldness. Besides, I felt more and more that I had less and less to hide. While I was absent from the judges' common room in Vereeniging, Judge-President Eloff must have mentioned to colleagues that I wasn't well. (And why should he not?) Colleagues began calling me at home. How was I? Could they do anything to help? They were missing me at court. I should get well soon.

My family's love and that of many friends had always felt secure. But it began to dawn on me that there was much, much more support and acceptance available to me than I had realised. And that I could draw on it. My anxious fears about my colleagues' possible reactions to AIDS began to yield to the loving reality of collegial acceptance and support. Of course they didn't know (or didn't know for sure) that it was AIDS. But some of them surely guessed. And in any event the fact was that it didn't and shouldn't make a difference.

After six weeks of feeling seriously sick, I was no longer in any mood to footle around with discrimination in the judges' medical insurance scheme. By Africa's standards, my salary was indeed comparatively large. But needy dependants in my household and outside it shared it with me. And I could simply not afford to continue spending one-third of my total disposable income on the new drugs.

Towards the end of November, after my ten days off, we resumed in Vereeniging. During a short adjournment, while police witnesses were being summoned to court, I opened my laptop. Spurred on by new energy and new determination, I wrote my judicial colleague a swingeing account of my sustained entreaties to him. Yet, I charged, he had delivered on none of his promises. If he was not willing to take immediate action to end the irrational discrimination against AIDS, he should, I suggested, resign from the medical scheme's board.

For good measure I wrote also to Judge-President Friedman of the Cape, a wise and humane man who had had originally been responsible for securing my colleague's appointment to the insurance scheme's board. The reaction of both was immediate – and positive. Expressing warm concern, Judge-President Friedman invited me to meet him in his chambers in Cape Town during the December vacation. I arrived fully prepared for confrontation with my dilatory colleague. Instead, he too was all readiness to help. Both he and Judge-President Friedman undertook that the matter would be dealt with properly and immediately. The unfair anti-AIDS discrimination would be set right.

And in the new year it was. The judges' and parliamentary medical insurance scheme stopped discriminating against AIDS as a chronic medical condition. First it granted AIDS the same coverage that all chronic medical conditions received. Later it increased its coverage for all AIDS conditions and treatments even more. Currently it offers judges and parliamentarians more than ample support for antiretroviral treatment – at least, for those judges and members of the legislature who are willing and able to claim its benefits.

In the meantime, the court year was drawing to a close. My colleague in the case of the young insurance fraudster called me to say that he had thought further about the case. He was now more convinced than ever that the magistrate's sentence was correct. I took the opposite view. Further reflection had made me conclude that the magistrate's sentence was wrong, and that our intervention was required. It became clear that we would not reach agreement on the outcome on whether the young man should be given a second chance. Because of our deadlock, Judge-President Eloff had to convene a new panel to hear the appeal again. He presided himself. Two other judges sat with him – three in all, so that if they too disagreed, the majority would prevail. Although the new panel also hesitated, the three judges all decided that justice required that the young man be given a chance to make good. He would not go to jail. He would keep his job. And he would repay the insurance company benefit payout that he had falsely claimed. He, too, would have a second chance. A sentence hanging over him – admittedly, not a death sentence – would be remitted.

My week-long break had come to an end. Again I started the daily drive to Vereeniging. But by then I realised that something incontrovertibly extraordinary was happening with my body. I was taking all my antiretroviral tablets twice a day, observantly and carefully. It certainly was not a breeze. The protease inhibitors in particular were difficult and unpleasant. The tablets were bulky and hard to swallow. At room temperature the precious drug soon degraded and lost its efficacy. The plastic capsules became blistered and started bleeding their contents. So they had to be kept chilled at all times – for the eighteen months I took them – making travelling very complicated.

What was more, the protease inhibitors left an utterly vile taste. Two hours after taking them, morning and evening, my stomach would erupt in gastric protest. For months after starting on them, I battled nausea. I also developed what the doctors call 'peripheral neuropathy' – nerve endings that responded badly to the new chemicals in the body. In my case, the nerve response manifested as peri-oral neuropathy. My teeth and sinuses became intensely and painfully sensitive. I remember coming into the kitchen one morning and biting into what seemed a deliciously tempting watermelon slice someone had left out of the fridge overnight. The room-temperature contact caused me to wince and then weep with pain. It was far too cold for my agonisingly ultra-sensitive teeth.

But all this was trivial beside the growing realisation that something quite unmistakably dramatic was taking place within my body. My tiredness was lessening. It was disappearing. In its place, I could feel a daily access of miraculous new energy. Life forces were coursing through my body. Illness was yielding to a nearly novel feeling – renewed and joyful wellbeing. Every evening, every morning, every long court day in Vereeniging, as I heard evidence in court, evidence of a different kind presented itself to me through my body. It was there – in the way my blood coursed through my veins, the way I heard myself breathe, the way my muscles felt. I not only regained my appetite – despite the nausea the protease inhibitors induced when I took them, I became ravenously and continuously hungry. For the first time in months, my stomach was digesting food properly. And my gaunt body avidly claimed every morsel of it to make up for the twelve kilograms (twenty-five pounds) in weight I had lost.

There was only one word for it. It was glorious. The drugs were working. I could feel that I was getting healthy again. I knew that I would be well again. That, in turn, spurred my inner confidence. Physiological wellbeing had a pronounced psychic effect. If the drugs were working – and it was utterly clear that they were – it meant that for the first time since my infection more than twelve years before, the virus was no longer multiplying within me. It was no longer progressively taking over my body, taking over my life. It was being beaten back to some deeply secluded (although still latently dangerous) viral reservoirs. But outside those recesses the rest of my body was free of it. And my immune system was, for the first time in all these years, free of its burdens.

The feeling was exhilarating. For the first time in more than a decade I was no longer – no longer felt – contaminated. From the world I had little to hide, and less to fear.

In December, just days after the meeting in Judge-President Friedman's chambers, my computer analyst sister Jeanie, her scientist husband Wim, and their two children joined me for a few days in Cape Town. After my original HIV diagnosis in 1986, I made a secret promise to myself – while they were young I would offer each year to take my niece Marlise and nephew Graham for a short pre-Christmas holiday in Cape Town. The beneficial delight in the beaches, long drives, silly vacation movies and chatter was, I always suspected, more wholly mine than theirs. The glorious Cape sun always blessed us with indolence. It was perfect rest. But each year we did one incontestably strenuous thing. We climbed Table Mountain.

Perhaps one of the best-known sights in the world, the sandstone massif dominates Table Bay. For hundreds of years, since Sir Francis Drake's voyage around the world, the view of it and the view from it have arrested travellers, justly evoking lyrical descriptions. The whole mountain is now a nature reserve, jealously guarded by Capetonians and the conservationists and researchers from all over the world who treasure and study and walk amidst its priceless floral and faunal heritage.

The mountain rises 1 000 metres above sea level, its sheer rock faces hundreds of metres high. From a distance, the famous 'table' front looks like a monolith of rock. It is not. The frontal rock is deeply split by a gorge that angles across and into its face. Platteklip Gorge is a particular hikers' favourite, and one of the best-known routes to the top. In the 1940s Churchill's ally, South African Prime Minister Jan Smuts, favoured it for his regular walks.

We decided to tackle Table Mountain. On International Human Rights Day, 1997, early on a startlingly sunny morning, we started the ascent. My brother-in-law, Wim, was not as keen as the rest of us. But with an accustomed family mix of infectious enthusiasm and browbeating coercion we persuaded him to join us. Little did we know how well-justified his reluctance was. Two days later he was diagnosed with acute appendicitis and had to be rushed into hospital for emergency surgery.

But at the time no hint of illness of any nature seemed to mar the day. The path up Platteklip Gorge begins at a fresh reservoir of mountain water. As we set out past it I wondered whether I would make it to the top. Just seven weeks before I had not been able to climb forty steps from the common room to my chambers. Now, cleared of the PCP and with the virus incapacitated by four weeks of effective antiretroviral therapy, I proposed to tackle more than eight hundred steps up the face of Table Mountain.

Jeanie and Wim stopped often to check on me. Was I making it? Yes, I was. Not without effort. Not with any speed. But I was making it. Twice the path crosses the stream that feeds the reservoir below. Then it heads steeply into the gorge that splits the sandstone cliffs. I drank deeply, thirstily, from the stream each time. The proteas, ericas, disas and pelargoniums that line the path, magnificently casual in their beauty under the mild December sunshine, seemed to beckon me up and on.

As we reached the top we paused, relieved and exhilarated, before strolling to the cable station restaurant 500 metres away across the flat rock plateau. As so shortly before, the climb had made me breathless, panting and sweating. But this time it was with exuberant joy. I knew that I was well, could be well, would be well. I had been given a second chance. As I gasped in the mountain air, I also knew what a mountain of privilege had brought me there. There was much work to do.

2 | Just a virus, just a disease

AIDS is a disease. It is an infection, a syndrome, an illness, a disorder, a condition threatening to human life. It is an epidemic – a social crisis, an economic catastrophe, a political challenge, a human disaster. AIDS is known. It has been analysed assessed assayed tested measured surveyed considered reflected documented depicted exhaustively described. Its virus is primal particular sub-cellular mutant enveloped nitrogenous. Our knowledge of it is clear and precise. But the disease is also unknown. It is guessed estimated projected approximated sketched debated disputed controverted hidden obscured. Still, it is mere fact: an event, a circumstance, a happening, a reality as present as the ocean or the moon.

AIDS is mouth and tongue and scar and nerve and eye and brain and skin and tum and gut. AIDS is smell and feel – of sweat and grime and snot and breath and bowel and secretion, discharge, pus, putrescence, disintegration, excrement, waste. Human waste. AIDS is feeling – painful sharp tingling burning heavy dull weakening wasting enervating diminishing destroying bereaving. AIDS is fear. It is breathless and nameless.

AIDS is stigma disgrace discrimination hatred hardship abandonment isolation exclusion prohibition persecution poverty privation.

AIDS is metaphor. It is a threat a tragedy a blight a blot a scar a stain a plague a scourge a pestilence a demon killer rampant rampaging murderer. It is made moral. It is condemnation deterrence retribution punishment, a sin a lesson a curse rebuke judgment. It is a disease.

AIDS is a disease triggered and sustained by a virus. The virus is the most researched and best understood in the history of humankind.

Scientists know precisely how it is genetically constructed and how it is chemically made up. We know how HIV replicates, how it is transmitted, and how it works to destroy the body's defence mechanisms, causing the catastrophic breakdown of immunity that is AIDS. We know a great deal about how HIV moves through populations and what social factors hasten its spread. We also know what living conditions and social circumstances speed up the onset of AIDS after someone has been infected with HIV. AIDS is the most scrutinised and studied and analysed disease in the history of medicine.

Even so, there is much that is unknown. Some continuing puzzles concern its epidemiology (the study of the spread of disease). We don't know exactly how many people are infected with HIV, or the precise number of those who have died of AIDS. For some areas, like North America and Australia, the figures are almost exact and very reliable. In other regions, those that AIDS most heavily burdens, the figures are estimates – for the most part, very rough estimates. These are based on well-established methods of inference and models of disease projection. But their application and the results derived from them are rightly the subject of a good deal of controversy.

Other puzzles are concerned with how the virus itself operates and how the human body responds to it. Some individuals, a tiny fraction, remain uninfected despite extensive exposure to HIV. We don't know why. Others, also a miniscule number, remain free of illness despite long infection with HIV. We are not sure why. Some populations have escaped the mass infection patterns that signal an epidemic. Others, in central and southern Africa, have not. The reasons are not clear. Anyone who pretends to know exactly why is pretending.

AIDS is the worst microbe-borne epidemic since the great plague, probably carried by rats and passed on from their fleas to humans, killed at least 25 million people – one third of Europe's population – in the mid-1300s. At least the same number of people have already died from AIDS. The United Nations special agency dealing with the epidemic, UNAIDS, estimates that by the end of 2002, after the epidemic's first two decades, cumulatively 25 million people had died from AIDS. In 2002 alone, as many as three million people died. The same agency estimates that there are currently more than 42 million people worldwide living with HIV or AIDS.

AIDS was first diagnosed in North America. But most of those whom AIDS now threatens with death live in Africa. Africa is the world's poorest continent. In the last five hundred years it has suffered the ravages of slavery, colonialism and exploitation. It continues to be crippled by debt and by the exclusionary policies of the world trade system, enforced by wealthy countries, which exclude its products from many profitable markets while undercutting the prices its farmers can obtain for their produce. Currently perhaps as many as thirty million Africans have HIV or AIDS.

The most signally important thing about AIDS is a hopeful fact – that it can now be medically managed. When the virus's replication within the human body is disabled, its effects become remediable. Drug treatment can now stop viral replication. AIDS is therefore a manageable condition. The drugs that disable viral replication exist, in ample number and manifold combinations. They are capable of being produced cheaply. What prevents their inexpensive production and ready distribution is in the first instance laws, national and international, that protect the exclusive rights of the corporations that have intellectual property title (patent rights) to them.

Where the drugs are available and accessible, and are administered under proper medical management, AIDS illnesses and deaths have been reduced by as much as 90 per cent. This has happened in affluent areas of the world. The epidemic therefore confronts business and political leaders with a pressing moral question. The means to prevent death from AIDS exist. Are they willing to take the measures needed to ensure that adequately supervised treatment reaches thirty million Africans and other people in the resource-poor world – or will they let them die because they are poor?

This question is pressing because without access to the new drug treatments, most of the 42 million people in the world living with HIV and AIDS will die of AIDS over the next ten years. Death from AIDS is lingering, painful, and (particularly in resource-poor settings) very short of dignity. And because AIDS is a syndrome of disparate diseases – because unlike cancer or ailments of the circulatory system or heart it does not strike efficiently at a single vital organ, but allows wasting disorders gradually to wrack the body as a whole – and because most of those with AIDS are young adults whose bodies are otherwise still relatively strong, death from AIDS is almost invariably a ghastly, drawn-out event.

Perhaps worse than many of its other features, more puzzling, less tractable, and besides complicating everything else, AIDS is also shame.

Shame – the humiliation or distress that arises from self-knowledge of dishonour or offence or impropriety or indecency.

An apparently insignificant incident kept me thinking for a long time. On an early spring afternoon in March 1993, while I was visiting London on a government-sponsored information tour, my foreign office hosts set up a meeting with a British writer and AIDS activist whose work I particularly admired. I arrived at the National Gallery before our appointed time to catch a glimpse of some of my best-remembered images – the shadowy elusions of Leonardo's drawing of the Virgin and Child with St Anne and St John the Baptist, the wiry-haired alert little dog attending the betrothal of van Eyck's Arnolfini, the altogether more languid pooch enjoying the hot afternoon with Seurat's Bathers, and the twisted death's head soaring sombrely past the feet of Holbein's handsome Ambassadors.

Under the coffee shop's thickly barred windows overlooking Trafalgar Square, my companion and I seemed to establish a quick rapport. Although visiting as an 'anti-apartheid lawyer', I was familiar with his subtle but passionate criticisms of conventional responses to gay sexuality and to AIDS. He in turn expressed a sympathetic connection with the problems weighing on me – how to stem the disquieting rise in HIV infections at home while trying to lay the ground for wise AIDS policies by our soon-to-be-elected democratic government.

As our conversation ranged widely, I began to sense in my companion a personal passion about the issues that I not only admired but which seemed to resonate with my own. But this was suddenly abbreviated when he paused to say significantly: 'Of course commitment does not have to mean you are HIV positive yourself. For instance, I'm HIV negative.' I was instantly puzzled. The avowal seemed illogical, unconnected. It exuded cold breath over our conversation like a lump of dry ice on a stage. Naturally I accepted what he said at face value. But I felt dismay spreading from my throat. If he was HIV negative, why did he need to insist on it? Surely such a thoughtful and provocative activist should avoid divisive, self-exempting labelling? Our conversation foundered. He took the check and soon after we parted ways on the steps of the gallery in the chilly dusk of late winter.

When I returned to South Africa, I wrote to thank him. But I decided not to ignore his pointed self-labelling. So I added a question. Why had he declared himself HIV negative, I asked, when the struggle for justice surely required indifference within it between those who are positive and those who are negative? I never received a reply.

But a few months later I bumped into him at a meeting in Berlin. That may have been my answer. He looked shocking. He was haggard and drawn, severely stressed or very ill – or, I thought, both. Later a mutual friend told me he had fallen ill with AIDS. He was probably feeling the effects of his impending slide downwards when we met at the National Gallery. He survived for long enough to benefit from antiretroviral treatment. He continues to write, as sensitively and perceptively as before. That he knew he was HIV positive when we met at the National Gallery seems almost certain.

Why could he not tell me? More precisely, why did this nuanced, committed person feel that he needed to make an unsolicited claim that he was HIV negative? Perhaps he feared that I imputed a personal connection to AIDS. Perhaps the adopted reserve of the southern English made the conversation's intensity uncomfortable. Perhaps he envied the lawyerly detachment he imagined that I was bringing to the issues.

Or did he just feel scared and lonely, fearful that I would encase him in stereotype, one all too familiar in those years – the self-interested, angry, afflicted, imminently perishable AIDS activist?

Perhaps he was already ill. Perhaps he felt the crackling drag of death upon his will, his energy, his courage, his life, as mortality hovered. Perhaps like us all he thought that denial deferred death.

If he had been asked, my companion could perhaps have answered some of these questions. But they should more truly have been directed at myself. For what was equally telling about our meeting that afternoon was that I, too, did not speak about my own exposure to HIV. For at the time I, too, knew that I had HIV. For more than six years I had known, since a Friday afternoon in December 1986 when my doctor, a well-meaning family friend on the point of retiring from a much-loved practice in Pretoria, phoned me during a busy moment at the Wits University human rights centre to tell me, without precursor, planning, request or approval, that he had sent my blood for testing, and that it had come back positive for HIV.

I look now in my legal appointments diary for Friday 19 December 1986. Court was in recess. The day notes the address of a close friend who had recently relocated to Cape Town. It fixes a lunch date with a funder at a nearby health food bar at 12h15. And it lists an arrangement to take two friends to the airport at 16h00 for a family visit abroad. My doctor's call came just after three o'clock. It delayed me, so that I was late for my friends. Not because we spoke for long. We didn't.

My doctor seemed nonplussed – grave and somewhat lost for words. But after he put the phone down I felt too stunned to move, incapable of my own distress. Eventually I dragged myself up. My first duty in a new, irreversibly changed world. My friends and I battled to reach the airport through a crashing Highveld thunderstorm that whipped the Friday afternoon traffic. Somehow they made their plane, and I made it home.

What the diary does not show is that later that night, in the state of acutely heightened awareness that sudden shock or bereavement can bring, I visited a busy bar in Hillbrow, Johannesburg's cosmopolitan flatland. Standing in the crowd I felt not dulled but sharpened, uselessly so, my awareness not stupefied but concentrated, futilely, as though something intensely violative had befallen me, a limb suddenly torn off, for which no previous experience had prepared me and about which nothing could now be done. Alone in my car on the way home I operated the controls as if for the first time, the steering wheel unfamiliar beneath my palms. The silence around me seemed intense. All the organs through which I was breathing had suddenly been fixed with an unspecified but surely imminent term date.

The shock was double. Apart from the blow of learning that I was infected, most immediately I felt as though I had experienced a stunning bereavement – the impending loss of my own life. I was thirty-three, building my career. In many ways – developmentally rather than chronologically – I was just starting life. AIDS was incurable. Its eventual effects were horrific – and untreatable. In South African law, when an assault or road accident survivor sues the perpetrator, a separate heading under which compensation can be recovered – apart from the victim's claim for expenses, pain and suffering and loss of amenities – is for 'loss of expectation of life'. It is a bereavement the cold categories of the law recognise.

For the first time I knew what it meant to experience a loss of expectation of living. I knew with certainty that I would fall ill soon. And then I would die. Death would assuredly overtake me within a year or two. Even discounting these dramatic presentiments, AIDS put a short, sudden and shocking limit on my life. In December 1986 it was for me what for tens of millions of Africans it still is today – an imminent term of death.

Over the next ten weeks, through a stint at Harvard law school's human rights programme, the bruising sense of shock and the enveloping silence travelled everywhere with me. The east coast newspapers and the bleakly pessimistic gay press of early 1987 fed my sense of horror on a daily basis. They proclaimed the rising death toll, the horrific manifestations of AIDS, their certain culmination in death, the social revulsion the disease almost everywhere evoked. Again, this not unlike Africa today for those with AIDS – a sense of horror, mixed with fear not only of the disease's effects but of people's reactions to it: and above all absence of hope.

In my shock I experienced what I later gathered is not uncommon among those not fairly forewarned of an HIV diagnosis: a sudden onset of AIDS-like symptoms. As I left for Cambridge, Massachusetts, I had a severe chest infection, sore throat, swollen lymph nodes. These all presaged, albeit mildly, the illness's eventual onset more than ten years later: vivid proof of the conjuncture of mind and body.

From America, baffled by his conduct, I sent my doctor courteous notes, diffidently enclosing patient information pamphlets and medical journal articles. These enjoined doctors – for ethical, psychological, legal and practical reasons – to obtain a patient's fully informed consent before HIV testing. They emphasised that the patient needs help and support – counselling – to cope with the result, whether positive or negative. In no circumstances should the news be communicated by telephone. A support structure should be in place. Never, ever, should the patient be left to face the news alone.

In the more promising days of treatment access, these norms are swiftly changing, and rightly so. Where life-saving treatment is available to the patient, it may be the doctor's duty to push the patient gently to agree to be tested. In Botswana, South Africa's land-locked neighbour, President Festus Mogae's government in 2001 announced a far-seeing national plan to provide antiretroviral treatment through the public health service to everyone with AIDS. But, as the death toll from AIDS continued to climb, poor enlistment baffled government health planners. So from January 2004, the Botswana government announced that unless patients at public health facilities actively declined to be tested for HIV, the test would be routinely administered.

Some of my activist friends felt dubious about the change. I differed. Provided that treatment is available, with guarantees of confidentiality and against discrimination, I thought and still think that testing is more often than not necessary, and beneficial. It is better that health workers, trying to be true to their calling of beneficence, should nudge patients who may need treatment towards the HIV test than that they allow patients to return home, trapped by fear and stigma, untested, to add to the epidemic's already appalling toll of unnecessary deaths.

By contrast, where no treatment is available – as in the bleak 1980s, and as is still the case through most of Africa – testing may do little more than expose those who prove positive to stigma, ostracism and discrimination. And without proper support (including counselling) an unpresaged HIV positive test result is almost always damagingly counter-productive. So my doctor erred doubly. But looking back I have scoured my conscience to ask whether part of me in fact suspected that he might use my annual visit that year to test for HIV. Every year when I visited him in early December for a check-up, he sent blood for liver function tests and platelet counts and cholesterol – benign, incomprehensible checks that held no meaning for me and less fear. They always came back clear.

But AIDS in the mid-1980s was a burning issue for young gay men. Perhaps with all the current talk, with the previous year's Sunday headlines agog with news of the 'gay plague' that had reached South

Africa, with my doctor's knowledge of my sexually active post-divorce life . . . perhaps between thought and suspicion and expectation and hope it must have crossed my mind that he might also take it upon himself to test for HIV. But if I did conceive of such a decision at all, without his first discussing it with me, without arranging for counselling or for support or follow-up afterwards, it was only because I hoped and believed that those results, too, would be benignly insignificant.

Perhaps my doctor did too. But the positive result was all too comprehensible. It meant death. And I had had no preparation for anything so instantly and brutally terminal. I had no doubt that he should have consulted me first, and that he should, on getting the positive result, have arranged matters very differently. Neither privately nor professionally have I ever met a person, young or old, employed or unemployed, numerate or innumerate, literate or illiterate, housed in stone or brick or corrugated iron or plastic sheeting, for whom the significance of such a result is any different. Your state of health – the term of your life – is a matter of deepest privacy, most integral to your conception of your life and being. It is part of what defines hope and expectation. It has been said that what distinguishes humans from other animals is our conscious apprehension of mortality. That sense – its translation into present knowledge – must always be approached, addressed, its imminence determined and imparted, with utmost veneration.

No person, professionally qualified or not, ill-intentioned or well-meaning, for instrumental or intrinsic purposes, has the right to grasp that knowledge without at least first consulting and preparing the person it most concerns. That is more especially the case when the result reveals a reviled disease exposing the patient to dread reactions; and when the medical diagnosis can offer no present hope and intervention to the patient diagnosed.

My frozen half-gestures to my doctor sought to communicate some of this. One emotional evening in early 1987, shortly after returning from Harvard, I managed to confide in my friend and Wits law associate Carole Lewis, now a colleague in the Supreme Court of Appeal. But apart from her, I made contact with almost no one. I confided, after a time, in the person with whom I fell in love the next year. To a wise and patient private counsellor, and to a Wits doctor doing brave early work in the field, Professor Ruben Sher, I spoke. But not to family or troops of friends. I feared their reaction with a ghastly, sickening, isolating loneliness. For more than three years I lived with it solitarily, not quite alone in a treeless tundra of my own involuntary creation.

Practising law at the human rights centre was gruelling but engrossing. In July 1985 and again in June 1986 the apartheid government plunged the country into a state of emergency, proclaiming punitive legal measures that banned meetings, publications, protests and political activity. Communities long-established on their land were still being 'resettled' – forced off it in pursuit of the grand design of racial separation and subordination. Ramshackle 'nations' were still being fabricated as part of the grand plan of separating black and white, and were being declared 'independent' of the rest of South Africa. Fighters for the exiled African National Congress infiltrated their homeland. They targeted, with extremely rare exceptions, non-civilians exclusively. When captured, they faced trial for treason and murder. Scores of young white men who refused to be conscripted into the army were imprisoned as conscientious and religious objectors.

But despite increasing depravities, for the most part the apartheid authorities still took the law and legal processes seriously. Court challenges often alleviated or obstructed the noxious and futile apparatus of racial subjugation. And it created spaces for trade unions to grow and flex their worker power. No day was dull. While work was sometimes dispiriting and often overwhelming, more often it was exhilarating.

It was also a diversion, a justification, a comfort and a distraction.

But it was not merely awareness of radically truncated mortality that seemed to be freezing my responses from within. Nor was it only fear of others' reactions to my condition. More horrifying was the inner sense of contamination I experienced. Yes, I felt too fearful to speak with anyone. But I also felt too ashamed. I was tainted, soiled, polluted. My blood and body were fouled with the most conspicuously vile infection known to recent human history.

Widespread and much publicised revulsion to AIDS – and fear of those with HIV – didn't help to combat these feelings: the witch-hunts at American primary schools, the rash of criminal legislation targeting those with HIV, the seclusion camps in Sweden and Cuba. In South Africa, proposals were mooted but fortunately abandoned, to force doctors to report cases of HIV or AIDS to the public health authorities. In August 1986, the mine bosses' organisation, the Chamber of Mines, announced the results of a study on blood samples of 300 000 male mineworkers. These showed that about 800 mineworkers – 760 of whom were from central Africa, in particular Malawi – had HIV. The reaction was drastic. The workers with HIV were summarily deported. This was achieved through the deadly mechanism of simply not renewing their yearly contracts at the beginning of 1988. Regardless of their years of service, they were sent back to Malawi – with its pitifully inadequate health system – to meet their fate.

It was this issue, brought to me because I was a human rights lawyer doing trade union work, that drew me into AIDS policy and litigation. Not my own condition, but a condition outside, graphically linked to apartheid injustice. It was easy to throw myself into AIDS activism in this guise. A dualism began. Publicly, I was a human rights lawyer involved with trade unions, community organisations, ANC fighters, military resisters – and HIV issues. Privately, AIDS was hideously, almost unthinkably, close.

Reactions like those that led to the expulsion of the Malawian mineworkers were all fuelled by a sense that those with HIV or AIDS had only themselves to blame. From this were excluded only the small minority of 'innocent victims' – children and blood transfusees, who could not be fixed with blame for their condition.

There is no doubt that many people thought and still think of those with AIDS or HIV as contaminated with a vile, self-induced affliction. But all too many sufferers are painfully conditioned into also thinking that way about themselves. Looking back on the problem I experienced in not being able to talk with my human rights lawyer colleagues, I see all too clearly that it emanated partly from within me. At some inaccessible, impenetrable level – even while challenging injustice against people with AIDS in the courts and on committees and on public platforms – I was still struggling with an overwhelming inner sense of shame. In some indefinable sense that I grappled to surmount, I felt that my infection showed that I had acted shamefully, dishonourably, so as to bring not only death but disgrace upon myself.

My colleagues were all committed – of course – to justice and fairness and nondiscrimination. But I confided in none of them. I could take no risks. Nor could I permit myself the comfort of connection. In dealing with clients and plotting public interest litigation challenges we developed close camaraderie and even friendship. But I could no more tell them that I had HIV than seek solace by confiding that I had molested one of their children or pets. That was how deep, how powerful, how repulsive my condition seemed to me.

Perhaps you think my reactions excessively subjective, or the comparisons overstated. But powerfully irrational responses to AIDS overshadow the epidemic even today. For stigma – a social brand that marks disgrace, humiliation and rejection – remains the most ineluctable, indefinable, intractable problem in the epidemic. Stigma is perhaps the greatest dread of those who live with AIDS and HIV – greater to many even than the fear of a disfiguring, agonising and protracted death.

Stigma manifests itself in hatred, discrimination, rejection, exclusion. Workers are sacked. Spouses are shut out. Friends are abandoned. Services, help and support are refused.

What is perhaps most poignant and most impenetrable about stigma is that some of its impact seems to originate from within. The external manifestations find an ally within the minds of many people with HIV or AIDS. Stigma's irrational force springs not only from the prejudiced, bigoted, fearful reactions others have to AIDS – it lies in the fears and self-loathing, the self-undermining and ultimately self-destroying inner sense of self-blame that all too many people with AIDS or HIV experience themselves. It is the combination of these two forces investing AIDS stigma that renders its effects so powerful and so destructive.

The external manifestations of stigma are horrific enough. At Christmastime 1998 a 36-year-old South African woman, Gugu Dlamini, was stoned and stabbed to death. The horror of her death has never been fully investigated, because her murderers were never held to account. The prosecution brought charges, but dropped them for lack of evidence. What is clear is that shortly before her death Gugu told Zulu-language radio listeners that she was living with HIV. Three weeks later, members of her own neighbourhood rounded on her. Her attackers accused her of shaming her community by announcing her HIV status. She died in hospital – her body broken not by the HIV she faced with such conspicuous courage, but by the injuries her neighbours inflicted on her. She left a thirteen-year-old daughter.

Three months after Gugu died I decided to announce publicly that I was living with HIV. My decision was impelled partly by horror at her murder. Simon Nkoli, a brave activist, died at almost the same time. His courageous openness about being gay while he shared a prison cell with other ANC leaders during the 1980s helped to ensure that gay and lesbian equality was included as a cornerstone of nondiscrimination under the democratic constitution. When he later fell ill with AIDS, Simon took the logic of confrontation and truthfulness a step further. He spoke out about the fact that he had AIDS.

He died, comatose, exhausted and dispirited, on 30 November 1998 – four days after his 42nd birthday. The new drugs had failed him. We surrounded Simon's body where it lay in the comfortless, busy wards of the Johannesburg general hospital. He had survived a childhood under apartheid – in the very Vaal townships near Sharpeville where a year before I had started my own quest for wellness on antiretroviral therapy. He had survived also a pitted, often fractured quest for love and friendship, and trial for his life on the capital offences of murder and treason. He did not survive AIDS. A media statement from family and friends stated his cause of death. More than six years after his death such openness, throughout Africa, still remains a rarity.

Simon's memorial service was held at St Mary's Anglican Cathedral, a capacious structure in downtown Johannesburg. Its traditional hewn-stone textures and spaces would not be out of place in the Cotswolds. It is here that the young Desmond Tutu, later Nobel Peace laureate, began his rise to prominence as a moral voice against apartheid's injustice. Over the unremitting decades of racial humiliation and subjugation, the cathedral served as the venue for many protests, many moving ceremonies.

Now Simon's coffin lay there. Somehow his obsequies seemed harder, bleaker, crueller. His life's struggle had helped create the South Africa to which Tutu aspired. Now he had succumbed to AIDS. On a rain-spattered, chilly Friday evening, despite the good turnout the cathedral felt skeletally empty. I joined the speakers who honoured Simon. I spoke about his dying from AIDS, about how signally important openness was in the struggle for acceptance and fairness. But still I could not speak about my own life with AIDS – a life sustained for more than a year now by the drugs that failed Simon – the drugs that continued to be denied to millions of South Africans and others who needed them.

Another brave anti-apartheid activist led the way for me. Three months before Simon died my friend Zackie Achmat broke his silence about living with HIV. In an emotional letter to his friends he spoke about his infection with HIV. Zackie is a man of immoderate intelligence, personal magnetism and courage. He combines these qualities with unequalled guile (the latter hard-learned on the streets and in prison as a teenage anti-apartheid activist) and a steely sense of strategy. Already he had energised gays and lesbians in our new democracy to unite in challenging discrimination under the new constitution. Now his openness seemed to inspire him with even deeper energies.

Soon after 'coming out' with his HIV, he launched the Treatment Action Campaign. Rapidly it became democratic South Africa's foremost activist organisation, shaming the international drug companies and challenging the government on many of its policies. It called on them to adopt comprehensive AIDS policies that would make the newly available drug treatments accessible to the millions of Africans who desperately needed them. Faced with years of collusive paralysis between international corporations and governments in Africa, the TAC confronted both with remorseless inventiveness – finely crafted legal challenges, superbly researched, principled arguments and uncompromising stands that often exposed Zackie and its other leaders to personal risk.

By the time Simon died at the end of 1998, it was clear that the drugs had saved my life. Twelve months after the onset of fully symptomatic AIDS, I should have been in a harrowing terminal decline, with repeated, increasingly severe infections winnowing the flesh from my bones and the energy from my body.

Instead, I was fit and well and energetic. I was still taking protease inhibitors – by far the most powerful of the new drugs. Though their neural side effects (the excruciating facial pain and dental sensitivity) and the nausea had long passed, the gastric effects they caused remained drastic. After every dose (six chilled capsules twice a day) my bowels twisted in spasm. But together with the other two drugs their effect remained unmistakably dramatic.

As I was experiencing the first heady upsurge from the drugs at the end of 1997, I was asked to chair the governing council of University of the Witwatersrand. It is a heavy but engrossing and deeply rewarding task. It has taught me some of the sorrow and complexity of trying to run a major educational institution. But it has also brought me the rewards of working with researchers and administrators and thinkers of extraordinary integrity and ability and dedication – including a close working relationship with Wits's first black vice-chancellor, a brilliant and engaging mathematician named Loyiso Nongxa, who like me had gone to Oxford on a Rhodes Scholarship.

My new energies spurred me daily, when I awoke, as I did my court duties, as I went to chair sometimes arduous and exacting meetings at Wits University and for my other 'causes', and as I spent evenings with friends. My energy, my appetite, my wakefulness all crested bountifully upwards.

Perhaps the drugs failed Simon because of the way in which he had become exposed to them. Like others living in mortal fear of AIDS at the time, Simon took them as they became available – successively and singly. After his release on bail in 1988, well-intentioned friends from abroad started sending him parcels of zidovudine (AZT). He took it for a time. Then he stopped taking it, later perhaps starting again. As other antiretroviral drugs became available, he took them too – first one, then another, then a third. By the time he fell seriously ill with AIDS in the mid-1990s, his virus had learned to outwit each drug in turn, becoming resistant also to similar drugs in the same class. So when he started combination therapy the virus had mutated into complex enough forms to evade confinement. It raged through his body until it finally prevailed over his strength on 30 November 1998.

By contrast, I had never taken any antiretroviral before. Thanks to my homoeopath I had for more than six years not even taken a single antibiotic. My body was 'drug-naive'. So when I started the knockout combination a year before Simon's death, it worked as Dr David Ho and his colleagues had dreamed it would.

Simon's death underscored for me the particularity and the partiality of my minor physiological miracle. Above everything else, I was taking the drugs only because I could afford to pay for them – at their still excessively inflated 1999 prices.

Publicly, on platforms, in committees and in the media, I spoke about the imperative need to make the drugs more widely available. Their prices had to be reduced. The drug companies had to be less graspingly miserly in sharing the rights to produce them. They had to permit poor countries to import them cheaply from other manufacturers. African governments – particularly South Africa's – had to commit themselves to tackling the crisis with concerted energy and determination. But on each of these issues I spoke in only a partial capacity – as a lawyer, later as a judge, always as an AIDS policy buff. Of my own experience as someone who had survived severe illness with AIDS because I could afford the drugs that gave me life, I still remained silent.

Surely if I started speaking as someone myself living with AIDS, I would do so with greater moral force, more unchecked energy, better clarity about what had to be done?

It would be only a matter of time. I knew this. My illness in late 1997 was relatively well disguised from Johannesburg's close-knit legal community, because when I fell ill I was out of town on the Vereeniging circuit. Only my assessors, who sat with me on the bench and shared my judge's chambers during adjournments, saw how ill I was. Word nevertheless did get about. Why should it not? One of my assessors in those first oxygen-depleted, antibiotic-laden weeks at Vereeniging was the father of my lovely godson, Sizwe Mpofu. He expressed concern to Sizwe's mother, Terry, about how ill I looked.

When she called to find out how I was, my initial response was panic and fear.

And yet my friends and colleagues were concerned, and wanted to express their concern and support. Why should they not? It was I who was not yet ready to receive it. My internal feelings of fear and disgust and self-blame were still too strong. I disentitled myself from the help I was entitled to claim and to receive.

There was wider talk. A journalist from a Sunday paper made an appointment to see me in my chambers at the High Court. He had heard it said at a dinner party, he told me, that I was HIV positive. Would I not give my 'story' to him? 'Speak to me,' he urged. 'If you don't, other less sympathetic journalists are planning to run with it.' This I doubted. I knew that without a firm factual source, or direct confirmation from me, newspapers were likely to defer to South Africa's stern privacy laws.

His tone of implicit menace offended me, and I frostily declined. Undaunted, he asked me directly if I was HIV positive. I paused for a moment while I looked him in the eye. I hesitated. I would not lie. But what was I to say? Then I told him the fable of the King of Denmark. He, it was said, publicly wore the yellow Star of David to signify solidarity with his Jewish subjects under Nazi rule – and saved them, alone amongst the occupied European communities, from obliteration. 'In that sense,' I told him, 'of course the only answer I can or am willing to give you is that I am HIV positive.' He published nothing.

The King of Denmark's tale was doubtless apt. But my response gaped incompleteness. And more important, from a personal point of view, it was utterly unsatisfactory. Gugu's death marked a terminus to this. It was a particularly poignant and sobering challenge. Bereft of the privileges of job and medical care, defencelessly exposed to a community that later turned on her, she nevertheless spoke out about her HIV.

By contrast, I was surrounded by protections and privileges. My job was constitutionally secure – unless two-thirds of Parliament voted to remove me, I could not be sacked. Behind my suburban wall I lived in relative comfort. Those of my friends and family and colleagues in whom I had confided offered me only love and support. And unlike Gugu I had the best medical care. I had life.

If Gugu could speak out, how could I not?

This question challenged me. It also unnerved me. But I accepted the only possible answer to it. The problem was – how? How to do it, where to do it, with whom. And above all how to minimise the risk of wrong-headed sensationalism? How could I speak truthfully about my own position while trying to place the focus on the millions who, unlike me, did not have the protections that might enable them to speak out?

This question I pondered with my activist friends. Earlier I had spoken to writer Mark Gevisser, with whom I had edited a book of essays on gay and lesbian lives in South Africa. Should I do it through a media statement, a news conference, an exclusive interview with a trusted journalist? Wisely, he gave his views on all these possibilities – but suggested that the circumstances would present themselves.

And indeed, this is what happened. A respected judge on the Constitutional Court, John Didcott, died after a long illness. The vacancy for his position was advertised. By the closing date for applications, I was the only candidate nominated. But the constitution required the commission dealing with the appointment of judges to place a shortlist of at least four names before President Mandela. So the closing date was extended, and more nominations were canvassed.

The commission would have to hold public hearings. They were scheduled for shortly after Easter. I faced a public interview – nothing exceptional, since I had appeared previously before the commission. But this one would prove to be different. On Easter Saturday the head of the Constitutional Court, Justice Arthur Chaskalson, suggested that I come for lunch at his home. In the 1980s he had spearheaded legal challenges to apartheid. Formidably intelligent and steely-principled, he was a mentor to many human rights lawyers. I trusted and admired him.

So when I was agonising over my HIV status on being nominated as a High Court judge in 1994, I confided in him. I went to see him in his chambers at the new Constitutional Court's temporary premises. His face registered shock and distress as I told him that I had HIV. But he quickly absorbed the implications – and concentrated on helping me with my dilemma: should I tell the judicial appointments commission? I was in good health. My immune system checks were at that time still looking good. I still believed and hoped that I might never fall ill, or at least that illness could be postponed for fifteen or twenty years.

We talked through the issue. He agreed that it was neither necessary nor appropriate to disclose my HIV status. With effect from 8 December 1994, President Mandela appointed me a judge of South Africa's High Court. A dream I thought would never be realised had been fulfilled.

So once before Justice Chaskalson and I had faced the issue of disclosure. I had also told him about the journalist's insinuating visit. And he had clearly given it thought. Almost casually in the course of our lunch he dropped the suggestion that I make a public statement about my HIV during my upcoming interview. As always, he approached the matter with strict rationality. 'There is nothing to be ashamed about,' he said. 'Many people have HIV. And the time has surely come for someone in public life to begin by speaking out. Why not simply do it at your interview in two weeks' time? The commission offers you an appropriate and dignified environment to do so.'

There could be no quibbling with his suggestion. What he'd said was logical and reasonable. And it was persuasive. It was clear that the time for which I had tried to prepare myself had arrived. But as we finished lunch and I left to drive home, I felt emotions heaving inside. What would friends and colleagues think? How would the press react? I would have to tell my 78-year-old mother, Sally. She had a vibrant circle of friends of her age. How would they respond? How would my sister and her family be affected? How would I feel on the street, amongst colleagues, walking into court, going into a bar or café? The inevitably sensational aspect of the event appalled and frightened me.

Overcome by apprehension, I stopped my car next to the roadside. For a while I leaned my head on the steering wheel and let grief overcome me. Afterwards I felt better. However awesome public disclosure seemed, Justice Chaskalson was right. What I proposed to disclose stood the test of truthfulness. It stood the test of usefulness. And looked at objectively there was no shame in it. Shame, in fact, my shame – other people's shame, our shame as people with HIV, the fear and inhibition that shame produces – was at the root of the problem.

My brother-in-law Wim and his family stoutly supported the move. So I set about telling close friends and colleagues who did not know. And on the Sunday before the commission convened I joined my mother for lunch at her retirement centre in the quiet Pretoria suburb of Arcadia. The autumn day was blissfully warm and sunny. In the early afternoon she and I took a slow walk through the lovely terraced gardens of the Union Buildings – the splendid sandstone crescent Herbert Baker had conceived in 1910 as the hilltop administrative hub of a white South Africa. Now the magnificent edifice proudly housed the offices of President Mandela and Deputy President Mbeki. Amidst the richly coloured cannas and late roses we sat down on a bench overlooking Pretoria's city bowl. I had to tell her that not only was I living with HIV – but that very shortly I planned to go very public.

But my mother had long followed my career. Always she expressed support and admiration for my work in AIDS. In my worst moments I had thought I would not survive her. Now I could truthfully emphasise how well I was feeling on the drugs. Our deaths, parent and child, would be in due order.

I brought the conversation around and spoke gently to her. When I had finished there was a quiet pause. She continued looking calmly, almost abstractedly, at the flowerbeds. After a moment she glanced at me, and quietly murmured: 'I thought as much, my boy.' Later that week, when Jeanie discussed the implications with her, she became distressed. But she started wearing the red, furled ribbon of AIDS solidarity. And her friends splendidly followed suit. She died two years later, ten months after we had celebrated her eightieth birthday. At her memorial service, I read out Zackie's evocation of her, 'always in your garden, always wearing her AIDS ribbon'.

The commission convened in Cape Town. I was the morning's first candidate. Zackie made sure that he was there, sitting just behind me. If he leaned forward he could touch me. That taught me something I had not quite experienced before about the tangibility, the felt proximity, the physiological closeness, that friendship and support can bring.

Justice Chaskalson introduced and welcomed me. He referred to my previous appearances before the commission – when I had been appointed to the High Court, to the labour appeal court, and a previous unsuccessful pitch for the Constitutional Court. The moment came. He invited me to read my statement 'about a personal issue you wish to entrust to the commission'. I began to read. My friends and I had carefully crafted it to deflect as much attention as possible away from the sensational angle some inevitably might take ('Judge has AIDS') to the material circumstances that made it possible for me to speak at all.

I emphasised that I had chosen to speak out even though legally and ethically I was entitled to remain silent. This choice was available to me 'for very particular reasons – because I have a job position that is secure, because I am surrounded by loved ones, friends and colleagues who support me, and because I have access to medical care and treatment that ensures that I remain strong, healthy and productive'.

Those three privileged conditions – a secure job in a nondiscriminatory environment, support of those closest around me, and life and health – were exactly what Gugu Dlamini deserved no more and no less than me, but was not privileged to have. We were particularly anxious that my statement should not expose others, unprotected as she had been, to unfair and premature pressure to be tested, or to reveal their HIV status.

'For millions of South Africans living with HIV or AIDS,' I went on, 'these conditions do not exist. They have no jobs, or their jobs would be at risk if they spoke about their HIV. They not only lack community support, but face grave personal danger if they do so. And, most importantly, they do not have access to proper medical care and treatment. For them, in a still hostile climate, the choices are strictly limited. Their right to invoke confidentiality remains of critical importance to them. It is only by creating conditions in which people can speak out without fear that we can begin to end the silence surrounding South Africans living with AIDS and HIV.'

I concluded by stressing 'my hope that my decision to speak today may contribute to a greater climate of openness and caring, and to the prospect of proper medical treatment, for all South Africans living with HIV or AIDS'.

For a few palpable moments the commission's judges, lawyers and politicians sat in stunned silence. I sensed that some of them had family – or feared they had family – who were closely affected. Perhaps their fears were closer still. Then the silence was broken by one, more, many questions. They seemed to embrace me, respectfully, supportively, even ardently. I emphasised that I had been able to choose to make my statement because 'I am not dying of AIDS. I am living with AIDS.' The phrase caught on.

Before, it had felt like the hardest, most self-exposing thing I had ever done. After, I knew that I had freed myself of a vast burden – that of unnecessary secrecy. I was able to unite myself with the truth, finally to disburden myself of responsibility for a secret that I had not wanted to keep. More deeply, I was relieving myself of responsibility for others' reactions to my illness. My silence was designed to forestall them from condemning, despising me. Now if they wished to condemn me, it was their decision. I no longer sought to control. After more than twelve years, it was an inexpressible relief.

And finally, the act of speaking addressed – for me at least – that unspoken shame at the core of so much AIDS discrimination. My silence entailed collusion between my inner sense of shame – however unjustified – and others' anticipated reactions of condemnation.

My act of speaking realised the simple truth in Justice Chaskalson's advice. There is nothing shameful about having HIV or AIDS. If we can talk about it, we normalise it. And the sooner AIDS becomes a normal disease, the sooner we will be able to deal with it unemotionally and effectively. Normally.

The commission lauded my statement. It recommended me for consideration by the president. In the end I was not appointed. The justice minister, Dullah Omar, a friend and colleague from cases and campaigns in the 1980s, telephoned me immediately after the cabinet meeting where the decision was made. He had been mandated, he told me, to emphasise to me how the cabinet had agonised over the choice. The post went to a highly respected High Court and labour appeal court colleague, Sandile Ngcobo. A tough-minded lawyer with wide experience and strong constitutional commitments, Justice Ngcobo had academic credentials in addition to practical experience. He had also trained in a Washington, DC law firm and in the chambers of United States circuit appeals judge Leon Higginbotham before returning to South Africa to work in public interest law.

He quickly established himself as a powerful force within the court. In a deserving twist of fate, he wrote the Constitutional Court's commanding opinion in the first AIDS case that came before it, Hoffmann *v* South African Airways. For me this suggested, as so often in my life, that events have their own timeliness, their own rightness, their own roundness.

The commission's favourable response to my declaration was a small foretaste of what was to come. Not only was the public and media response massively and generously positive, but journalists and editorial writers quickly developed further the notion that the silence about HIV could be broken only by creating the conditions of nondiscrimination in which people can feel free to speak out.

If positive reaction was not wholly universal, adverse reactions were extremely isolated. One parliamentarian in the largely white opposition party condemned me for bringing AIDS upon myself. His party resolved formally that he had to apologise – which he did, fulsomely, in a letter to me. A single newspaper commentator – coincidentally, also a white male – wrote sneeringly that it was hardly appropriate that I should seek to glory in my condition.

These were isolated voices. In both news columns and editorial comments, coverage otherwise was emphatically and expansively supportive. The welfare services minister, Zola Skweyiya, sent a huge flower arrangement with an affecting greeting signed from 'Zola and Thutha Skweyiya'. Only weeks before, they had suffered a terrible bereavement when their official chauffeur had accidentally killed their young son in a driveway collision at their home. Their words were heartfelt.

Another minister, Deputy Justice Minister Manto Tshabalala-Msimang, herself a medical doctor, wrote with particular warmth:

'My office wishes to add its voice amongst those,' she said, 'who have been deeply touched by your courage and selflessness in the disclosure of your HIV status. We believe this notable act will contribute towards greater awareness of the HIV/AIDS issue. We also believe that it will contribute towards greater acceptance and protection of the human rights of persons living with HIV/AIDS.' Neither writer nor recipient could know that within weeks she would be promoted to health minister in President Mbeki's new cabinet, but that her treatment of AIDS would be dogged by desperate controversy.

Many others, in the cabinet and elsewhere, followed suit. From all over Africa and the rest of the world I received hundreds of calls, letters, messages and emails.

My judicial colleagues also reacted well. The afternoon after my statement, I flew back to Johannesburg. In the evening, the news of my statement led with other stories on the main evening television and radio bulletins. As I drove to the court the next morning, posters lining the streets inevitably proclaimed 'JUDGE HAS AIDS'.

But when I opened the door of my chambers, flowers had arrived before me. An Afrikaans-speaking colleague, Pieter Schabort, whom I had always identified as conservative, was the first to come by. He popped his head around my door – 'Strength to you, my friend,' he said. 'We're proud of you.' In a sense the flowers still haven't stopped coming. Nor has the release of positive energy.

But stigma remains. It is intense and real and prevalent. When I made my statement, I was confident that within a very short time other African leaders would follow – cabinet ministers, entertainers, sports stars, Members of Parliament. This has not happened. In South Africa, President Mbeki's open scepticism about whether HIV causes AIDS froze many reactions. In a speech in Parliament in late October 1999, six months after he succeeded President Mandela, he began a three-year apparent association with AIDS denialism – the scientifically unfounded doctrine that attributes AIDS exclusively to social and behavioural factors, and not to the physiological (and medically treatable) effects of a virus.

Nowadays he rarely speaks about AIDS, leaving it to his deputy president and to the health minister, Dr Tshabalala-Msimang. Her statements unfortunately also appear to reflect scepticism that AIDS is virally caused and can be medically managed. President Mbeki has never publicly stated that he accepts that HIV causes AIDS, nor that AIDS can be treated with antiretroviral drugs, though in his state of the nation address to Parliament in May 2004 he gave welcome public endorsement to antiretroviral treatment options when he committed government to a target treatment figure by 2005.

But in the years following his October 1999 speech, the president's apparent scepticism about the viral aetiology of AIDS, and the resulting public controversy, brought a profound chill to the attempt to bring reason and calm to the debate about AIDS policy in South Africa. It certainly seemed to stifle initiatives to openness about HIV that others in public office may have contemplated.

Certainly within South Africa, stigma has remained stubbornly intransigent. It would be crass to blame political attitudes for this when, as became evident to me, the roots of stigma lie so deeply within our own profound thoughts and feelings.

Partly because of stigma's continuing intransigence, the United Nations agency for AIDS, UNAIDS, proclaimed stigma its campaign theme for World AIDS Day 2003. It was a rightful focus. Stories from Botswana – a prosperous and cohesive southern African democracy squashed shoulder to shoulder between South Africa and Namibia – tell a sobering tale about stigma. Until recently many people seemed willing to face suffering and even death rather than receive help.

About one third of Botswana's people have AIDS or HIV – perhaps two-fifths of all young adults between 15 and 49. The government with unstinting forthrightness accepts the extent of the problem. President Festus Mogae has warned that his nation faces what he bluntly calls 'extinction' unless the epidemic is properly handled. Government AIDS policies are well directed and clear. Officials are committed to their implementation.

These policies are not just the usual African mix of public awareness, counselling and prevention. They go dramatically further. In his national address in 2001 President Mogae made a breakthrough announcement. Together with international drug companies and the Bill and Melinda Gates Foundation, his government would offer treatment with life-saving drugs to every citizen with AIDS. It was a visionary and far-reaching commitment. It set a bold standard that other countries in Africa have now begun to follow (in May 2004, Malawi, one of Africa's poorest countries, announced its own $196 million programme to distribute free antiretroviral treatment to all who need it).

The Botswana government's pioneering commitment was widely known throughout the country. Yet takers were initially perilously few. One survey suggests that to stay alive and well more than 100 000 people in Botswana need the drugs without delay. Yet by late 2003 only about 15 000 people – perhaps fewer – had come forward to accept the free medication.

Why? I asked my hosts this question in June 2003, when I joined Botswana judges and business, civic and government leaders at an AIDS awareness meeting in Gaborone. President Festus Mogae had originally agreed to come, but was called away to a United Nations meeting in New York. He sent a well-liked and senior cabinet minister instead. She read his letter of apology. It had the ring of personal authorship. Despite severe (and audible) flu, the minister herself braved the Kalahari winter cold to attend. 'That's how important this issue is to us in the government,' she told the audience to applause.

My Botswana hosts gave me a one-word answer to my question: stigma. People are too scared – too ashamed – to come forward and claim what their government is now affording them as their right: the right to treatment, the right to stay well, the right to stay alive. The main medical centre in the capital, Gaborone, is the Princess Marina Hospital. The AIDS clinic here dispenses the treatments. Plans to allow doctors and nurses at private clinics to give the drugs to AIDS patients are being discussed. But they have not yet been implemented. So for now, poor people who need government-supplied drugs in or near Gaborone must go to the clinic at Princess Marina. Many of them – most still, it would seem – are deeply reluctant to do so. This, my hosts told me, is because they fear they will be identified as having AIDS. So they postpone it for as long as possible. They fall sick first. Even then they delay. They eventually go and stand in the clinic's queues. But mostly they do so only when they are approaching the point of death.

This led the Botswana government to introduce a radical re-think of HIV testing policies: wisely, I thought and still think (though some activist friends differ), from 2004 doctors in public clinics would test patients for HIV unless they expressly refused.

This change of policy, against the background of the offer of real treatment options, helps patients too fearful to confront their own HIV to be given treatment. Unless prompted, as in my own case, they all too easily postpone, prevaricate, suppress, deny. In dwindling hope and growing fear, they rationalise the symptoms they experience, dreading the diagnosis they fear they will eventually get. In some horrifically constrained sense, they are 'choosing' to die, rather than face the stigma of AIDS and find treatment. Illness and the attendant risk of death feel less horrific to them than the stigma of having AIDS.

That sense is internally, and not only externally, fuelled by the shame that many people with AIDS or HIV feel about their own condition.

And not only poor people fear what will happen if others think they have AIDS. A revealing moment in the minister's speech in Botswana in July 2003 showed her own fear. She told the audience how sick she had been all week. She wished us to know what an effort she had made, and how vital the issue was to her, her cabinet colleagues and to President Mogae. So sick had she been that she had cancelled all her other appointments – except this one.

Here she paused. She seemed to reconsider. Perhaps she realised that her story might cause her audience to wonder what exactly had kept her in bed all week. But she wouldn't let them jump to the wrong conclusions. So she looked up and pointedly added: 'I want to assure you all I only had the flu. That was all. It was only flu.'

The audience shifted uneasily. There was some laughter. But the chuckles seemed to stem less from amusement than from recognition of her anxiety, the laughter designed to allay it and to reassure her: we know why you are anxious . . . we understand and share your anxiety that others should not suspect you of having AIDS . . .

I winced. Some others I think did too. The incident in the National Gallery in London sprang to mind. Did she have to spell out that it wasn't AIDS? She certainly thought she had to. But why? She would not lose her job. By every principle President Mogae had publicly and repeatedly emphasised, that was unthinkable.

Perhaps she feared something worse – that we would think less of her – would despise her, hold her in contempt, or ridicule, for having AIDS or HIV. Her disavowal seemed to play right into the perception that having AIDS was something unworthy, disgusting, unclean, improper. But it stemmed from a sense within her. A sense shared by all too many people with AIDS or HIV.

My Botswanan ministerial hostess's attitude remains widespread. In the whole of Africa not a single elected official from any national parliament has stepped forward to say that he or she is living with HIV or AIDS. In a continent in which those with HIV or AIDS number in the many tens of millions, no cabinet minister or governmental leader has come forward to say: 'Yes, I too am living with this condition.'

Shortly before Botswana, I travelled to Zambia for a workshop with judges and magistrates and lawyers. In his opening address, Chief Justice Ernest Sakala movingly expressed the extent of Zambia's national tragedy. His personal backing and stature ensured that almost all his colleagues on the Supreme Court, together with most of the High Court judges, attended. He spoke plainly: 'The devastating effects of HIV/AIDS have not spared the Bench,' he said. 'The saying that if you are not infected with HIV/AIDS you have at least been affected is true for all of us. None of us seated here can deny the fact that in our families we have each lost a loved one because of HIV/AIDS.'

Seated beside him, I looked up from my notes. 'In our families we have each lost'. His own family? His cousin? A niece, nephew perhaps? Aunt or uncle? Or a mother, brother, father, sister, wife? Perhaps a son or daughter? This was getting close. Uncompromisingly close. And the same applied to the families of every one of the dozen or more judges present?

Even though I had myself lost friends, close ones, seen people die, I felt moved by the candour and urgency of Chief Justice Sakala's statement. When at the end of the long day I took a wintry evening walk through the streets of Lusaka, a gentle, friendly, desperately poor city, strangers met my eye, greeting me with the courteous engagement that seems endemic to African culture. I knew that according to national prevalence rates perhaps one out of every five of the young adults I saw on the street had AIDS or HIV.

By simple average calculation, that made it likely that apart from me at least one other judge in the workshop also had HIV. After my talk, animated discussion followed. Some of the judges spoke of how essential it was to create a climate in which their colleagues with HIV could, like me, speak openly. Yet no one did.

Why? To say that it is because of the enormous stigma still attaching to AIDS is to restate the problem. Why is there such stigma? Stigma often accompanies those diseases that are seen as incurable, deadly, transmissible and disfiguring. But it seems to mark most severely those conditions where the affected person is seen as responsible for getting the disease.

AIDS fits all these categories. As the new drugs become increasingly available, the stigma from incurability will surely wane. (That is why I think the Botswana government initiative on testing is so wise.) As more and more people are diagnosed and speak out, the stigma from silence will also wane.

But there remains something even harder to grapple with. The most inaccessible, the most intractable element of stigma is the disfiguring sense of shame that emanates from the internal world of some with HIV or AIDS. This sense colludes with external stigma, overcoming efforts to deal with the disease rationally, keeping those with AIDS or HIV in involuntarily self-imposed isolation, casting a pall of contamination and silence over the disease.

What causes this shame? I don't know. Without special expertise in behaviourism, psychology or the human soul, I can only cast within myself for some inkling of the truth. And my conjecture, neither novel nor dramatically revealing, is that it is to do with HIV and sex. HIV is a sexually transmitted infection. Perhaps other sexually transmitted infections leave similar feelings. I do not know, since (perhaps ironically) the only one I have ever had is HIV. That has been my fortune, where life's forces have taken me.

Why does sex leave shame? Perhaps it lies in the embarrassment that arises from exposure of what one thought was utterly private and intimate. Perhaps to admit to having a sexually transmitted infection is to be caught out in an act of sexual intimacy, with all its attendant embarrassment – and shame. Pregnancy, too, is a sexually transmitted condition. Women made to wear the scarlet letter in the darker days of sexual oppression might have experienced a comparable sense of shame. But pregnancy is a condition, not an infection. A pregnancy, even one unwanted, even one deemed illicit, holds life and hope and the possibility of growth and fullness. Infection with HIV offers none.

Certainly for me some of the internal shame seemed to come from the fact that my HIV came from a sexual act. In my case it was male to male penetrative sex. When my doctor told me that I had HIV that Friday afternoon in 1986, I was a gay man recently come out. Though always, in my practice and social and political life, I expressed myself as resolutely open and proudly gay, perhaps my sense of shame derived from the fact that my virus was homosexually transmitted. Or so I thought.

But this was wrong. As the African epidemic took hold and spread, it became clear that I was not alone. For millions of heterosexual Africans with AIDS or HIV it is no different. Their shame about HIV is as intense. Even women who say that they married as virgins and remained monogamous within their marriages express shame at their condition, and experience the difficulty of speaking out about having HIV.

Perhaps therefore the internal stigma is connected with the merely sexual – not homo- or heterosexual. Perhaps in our deepest selves we feel that a sexually transmitted infection shows others that we have been 'caught out'. The infection leaves a mark, a stain, a print, linking us back to an act so private, so intimate, so sacrosanct, so emotionally and spiritually unguarded – the moment of sexual coupling – that its external manifestation in an illness, its exposure to the world, is deeply embarrassing and therefore shameful.

Perhaps we still regard ourselves as guilty of some sort of sin of sexual contamination, as marked by moral inferiority, by an uncleanness or exposure of body, and hence a sense of moral inferiority. Some religious moralists inflame all this. They forget that AIDS is a disease. We all do.

These speculations remain painful. And they remain close to me. They must to any South African living in this fearsome, fearful epidemic. In my own household I experienced the telling force of stigma and shame. My garden was tended twice a week by a gentle, smiling man in his mid-thirties. 'Gladwell' (as I shall call him) loved its beds and corners and the two kitties and two ducks who share it with those of us who live there. My housekeeper's young daughters, Diana and Paulina Kekana, who share the property with me, would follow Gladwell around as he weeded and planted and mowed on Mondays and Thursdays. Over the eight years he worked for me I thought I came to know him well.

At the end of 2000 I saw his health declining. Worried, I asked him about it. Had he seen a doctor? 'Yes,' he said, 'I have been to the hospital. The doctor has given me pills.' 'But did he tell you what's wrong with you?' 'Yes, he says it's TB [tuberculosis].' This was plausible. For a few months it was. Until it became clear that the 'pills' Gladwell said that he was taking were not working. Gladwell was looking tired, becoming thinner. I decided to broach HIV with him. It was long after my own public statement, and Gladwell knew – he had seen – that the drugs had saved my life. More than most people in the country, I enjoyed contacts and access that would ensure drugs for him, if he wanted them. This he also knew.

I took him aside one day.

'I want to ask you: have you had an HIV test?'

'Yes, I have.'

'May I ask what the doctor said?'

'It was clear.'

'Are you sure?'

'Yes.'

'You know that I can help you, Gladwell.'

'Yes, I do. It was clear.'

'But you don't seem to be getting better. Are you taking your TB pills?'

'Yes I am.'

'Why are they not working?'

'The doctor says I must take them for another few months. Then I will be clear.'

I was sceptical. But how could I override what he told me? Zackie, who uses my home as a base when he is in Johannesburg, asked Gladwell the same questions. He offered to take Gladwell for an HIV test. He repeated the offer to get drugs. Gladwell refused. As he grew thinner, I had to relocate to Bloemfontein, where the Supreme Court of Appeal sits for almost half the year. When I returned at the end of May 2001, Sophie told me that Gladwell had returned to his family in Zimbabwe. At the end of June we received news that Gladwell would not return. He had died, five weeks after last tending my garden.

Did Gladwell die of AIDS? Probably. We cannot know. Gladwell did not want us to know. Yet, as I look back, I see things with greater clarity. I see that I failed Gladwell. My notions of autonomy and respect, so vital in principle, were misapplied in the lee of the jet fuel fires of fear and stigma and internal disentitlement that were consuming Gladwell's life. Although I thought that I was offering him help, and thereby the choice of living, in Gladwell's mind he had no choice. The stigma associated with AIDS left him no choice. Like those at the top of the World Trade Centre towers who 'chose' the horror of jumping one hundred stories to death, rather than the horror of being consumed by jet fuel flame, Gladwell 'chose' to refuse our offers of assistance. He 'chose' to return to Zimbabwe to die, rather than let us help him deal with AIDS.

Gladwell died of stigma and fear. Surrounded by fear and uncertainty, he made himself inaccessible to help. He was scared of stigma. But, more disastrously, I think he was also ashamed. Yet I could have done more to reach him. I should have done more to reach him. Looking back, I know now exactly what I should have done. Remorselessly, my conscience enacts it for me. I should have made an appointment with Dr Johnson – on a Monday or Thursday. I should have waited for Gladwell, and told him about the appointment. I should have told him that I was leaving for Dr Johnson in ten minutes. I should have told him he was free not to come. But I was going, and I wanted him to come – I wanted him in the passenger seat of my car. I should have opened the door and invited him to get in. I should have told him that my doctor would diagnose and if necessary treat him if it was AIDS. And that I would help him deal with his fears and loneliness if it was.

All these things I should have done. I did not. I failed Gladwell as much as stigma and the dislocation of his home country and southern Africa failed him. Gladwell is with me, in my thoughts, on my mind, in my reflections. He is with me more than comfort allows.

Looking back to the National Gallery, I can see a little more clearly why my companion and I parted in silence when we could have communed with each other about the fact that each of us had HIV. It was not the stigma of others that silenced us. It was our own. We had not yet accepted that AIDS is a disease. Perhaps we all still don't.

3 | Race, sex and death in Africa

AIDS is an epidemic enmeshed with sex and death. In Africa the epidemic is enmeshed with the politics of race and sex and death.

The most arresting character in Shakespeare's early drama about the politics of race and sex and death, Titus Andronicus, is not Titus, but the black man Aron, 'a Moor and the lover of Tamora'. Tamora is Queen of the Goths, brought captive to Rome but made Empress by the Emperor's sudden choice to marry her. She and Aron become illicit lovers. They bring into a world of white bigotry a black-hued child – 'as loathsome as a toad/ Amongst the fair-faced breeders of our clime'. All three end up doomed and damned. In a violent play filled with deceit and treachery and lust, Aron – 'his soul black like his face' – is no less violent and deceitful and treacherous and lustful than the rest. But in the final scene he shows himself also irredeemable. Condemned to an ignominious death as 'an irreligious Moor,/Chief architect and plotter' of the play's woes – the 'breeder of these dire events' – Aron at the end expresses only one dark regret: 'If one good deed in all my life I did/ I do repent it from my very soul.'

And through this all is woven Aron's race. The Emperor's brother is appalled that Tamora is having sex with 'swart' and 'barbarous' Aron. He warns her that Aron's 'foul desire' has made her honour black – the colour of her lover's body, 'spotted, detested and abominable'. But Aron is proud of his blackness. He derides his white antagonists, flaunting his sexuality. He 'mounts' the Queen, 'wantoning' with her. When Tamora's son rebukes him because he has 'undone' his mother, Aron brazenly ripostes: 'Villain, I have done thy mother.'

He throws back the racial imputations: 'Is black so base a hue?' A white skin is treacherous, since it will 'betray with blushing/ The close enacts and counsels of thy heart.' Aron's blackness is unblushing, assertively itself: 'Coal-black is better than another hue,/ In that it scorns to bear another hue.'

The themes of blackness, villainy and lust thread through Western literature and art, as they threaded through the white colonisation of Africa. Titus Andronicus comes vividly to mind because of a production I saw at Stratford-on-Avon in England's autumn of 2003. The black actor playing Aron filled the auditorium with unapologetic performance, dominating the stage with diction and body mass, making large the text's racial and sexual overtones. The production offered compromise on neither. Aron's bold rejection of the racism around him sank through the theatre, challenging the British audience to think contemporaneously. To me it also suggested a re-reading of Aron's confessional self-denunciation in the last act. Leaving the theatre, I suspected that the character's inflated self-execrations at the play's end must be ironic, a still-mutinous reaction to capture and subjection, the show trial self-immolation of one who despises his captors and the 'justice' they are inflicting on him. Beneath the excessive self-detestation, Aron remains defiant – and defiantly black. He throws his blackness back at his captors, a last bitter joke, playing into and showing up their prejudices: Shakespeare larger than his time, and larger than our own.

Shakespeare did not shrink from race or his awareness of race, or from the vile fact of racism. Nor did Mozart. Just a few months before the Stratford Titus, my London friends Timothy Dutton and Sappho Dias treated me to an evening in the stalls at the Royal Opera House at Covent Garden. In Mozart's enchanting opera, the Magic Flute, Schikaneder's libretto has a black Monostatos preying on the virtue of the captive Princess Pamina. The themes of darkness and light, black and white, damnation and redemption, richly fill the music and the libretto. But the opera is famously intricate, offering suggestive contradictions in its plot and symbolism.

This should discourage simplistic analysis of Mozart's treatment of black and white and race. Monostatos is indeed black, and he does prey on white Pamina. But in doing so he rails against the injustice and hypocrisy and prejudice of a world that requires him to for-swear love 'because a black man is hideous'. This is the bigoted white world's judgment Monostatos does not accept. Like Shakespeare's Shylock, he rebukes the racist preconceptions around him by asserting the obvious – he too is human: 'Have I not been given a heart? Am I not of flesh and blood? To live forever without a wife would be true hellfire. So, while I am living, I too want to caress and kiss and be affectionate. Forgive me, dear Moon, for I have taken as mine a white woman. White is beautiful, I must kiss her!' Doubtless the white moon is also imbued with white prejudices. In defiantly approaching Pamina, Monostatos warns her off: 'Should this cause you such grief, Moon, then close your eyes!'

Monostatos proves to be as unapologetic and unrepentant as Aron. His only crime is his wish to love. His conduct may affront his rank and betray the duty he owes to the Queen of the Night. But for him, his blackness is not and should not be an impediment to loving anyone, even a white princess. In an opera of richly suggestive ambiguities and nuances, Monostatos's unrepentant assertion of his blackness highlights the bigotry around him.

Yet the producers at the Royal Opera did not see it so. They seemed to fear that Monostatos's blackness would create offence. So at Covent Garden in 2003, unbelievably, a white man played Monostatos. But how did they deal with the libretto's central invocation of race? Simple. They cut it out. They excised the pivotal line 'weil ein Schwarzer haesslich ist – because a black man is hideous'. Incredibly, they took this line as an admission from Monostatos, instead of an accusation. So they airbrushed the racial challenge out of Mozart's great opera.

As a South African visitor to London I was baffled. And appalled. A rank history of racial oppression has forced South Africans, black and white, to confront their racial past. In national terms, we think racially – consciously, deliberately and obtrusively. We acknowledge the continuing presence of racial stereotypes and prejudices in too many areas of our nation's public and private life. Our constitution and our public codes expressly commit us to eradicating them. This doesn't mean that racism has gone away, or that you can overcome a racial past by ignoring it. There is too much evidence of persisting white prejudices and animosities for this. In turn this has sometimes made it possible for incompetent or malperforming public servants or business people to invoke race evasively by imputing racism to their accusers to cover their own sins of corruption or inefficiency. White racism in such cases spawns a racism-in-reverse; its evil legacy grows.

But racial oppression and racial subordination and racial preoccupations are a legacy the white settlement of Africa created, and it is one that all South Africans are struggling to eradicate. Pretending it isn't there is our least acceptable option.

The singer playing Monostatos in 2003 at Covent Garden gave a substandard performance. I was nevertheless a little surprised when the audience booed him at the curtain call. (I did not think English audiences had the mettle of Milan – or, on one occasion I witnessed, of Cape Town.) But I wondered how many that night might not also have been booing the producers' failure of truth in their presentation of Monostatos. To me it seemed typical of some attitudes in my own country that deny race and racial consciousness in confronting our history, and in planning for our future.

The producers surely deserved to be ridiculed for a craven but misguided attempt at 'correctness', one that erased any suggestion of nuance in Mozart's opera; one that missed Monostatos's angry rejection of white racism. Instead, they tried to erase the racial issue – and the prejudices still prevalent in Western Europe and Britain – by playing Monostatos white. The politics of race and sex and death reach no resolution through evasion.

Race and the epidemiology of AIDS collided in Africa in the 1980s. A rank colonial legacy of racial thinking and bigotry has plagued our understanding of AIDS in Africa. In the Western mind AIDS was first overwhelmingly a 'gay plague'. Until the mid-1980s its deathly way seemed to sear itself largely through the gay communities of North America and Western Europe. Studies on cause, transmission and treatment focused largely on gay men. But by mid-decade it was clear that there was also an African epidemic – one taking a strikingly different form from that in the West. By the end of 1986 epidemiologists knew that in transmission and effect the epidemic in

Africa was largely heterosexual. While in the United Kingdom the ratio of male to female cases was approximately 33:1 – only three females for every 99 men – in Africa that ratio was estimated to be one-to-one. Women were statistically as much at risk as men. For patent physiological reasons – because the woman in unprotected intercourse becomes receptacle to the man's semen – much more so.

In the middle of 1986 the British High Commissioner in Lusaka sent a despatch to the Foreign Office in London that described in horrific detail how, even then, the epidemic was cutting into Zambia's educated and ruling elite. Shortly after, Zambian President Kenneth Kaunda startled and moved many Africans in October 1987 when he placed on record that his own son, thirty-year-old Masuzyo Gwebe Kaunda, had died the previous December of AIDS. Kaunda addressed a poignant appeal to the world: 'It does not need my son's death to appeal to the international community to treat the question of AIDS as a world problem. We want to fight this together, regardless of who dies from it.' Reading for the first time about the British diplomatic despatch just months after my own visit to Lusaka for the judges' workshop, I wondered how much may have been lost between 1986 and 2003, when Zambian public life had at last attained the sort of openness that enabled its Chief Justice to state publicly that the family of every judge had suffered losses from AIDS.

The onset of the indisputably mass, heterosexual African epidemic in the mid-1980s sounded alarm bells in Europe and North America. Surely, public health experts and government officials reasoned, this must bode ill for them too? If in Africa, why not elsewhere? Those trying to manage the frightening scope of the gay epidemic reached a not illogical conclusion – that also outside Africa HIV would spread heterosexually. And they began to make not illogical projections – a mass epidemic could ensue. Prevalence rates in Europe and America, they began to predict, could reach those that some African states were seeing in the mid-1980s.

The British Parliament debated the impending mass epidemic at the end of 1986 in crisis mode. Official concern provoked media interest. Reports encouraged fears that a mass outbreak of HIV could occur, or was imminent. What the historian of the British response to AIDS has described as a 'mood of wartime emergency' swept the country. The tabloid *Sun* ran a feature, 'Have you got AIDS?' For its readers it featured a checklist of commonplace symptoms such as tiredness, weight loss and diarrhoea. This was more than enough to spark alarm, if not panic, amongst readers.

The London *Sunday Times*, which later gave credence to dissident theories on AIDS, ran a prominent series of articles that emphasised the heterosexual threat. Since risk was universal, the British government decided to act. A high-powered cabinet committee was formed. A national prevention and awareness campaign emphasised the dangers of heterosexual transmission. Early in 1987 leaflets were sent out to 23 million British households. There were advertisements in the newspapers, and 1 500 posters proclaiming. 'AIDS – don't die of ignorance'. Without doubt the campaign produced intense public awareness and high education levels about AIDS.

In America, too, alarm that the HIV epidemic would spread into the heterosexual community was pervasive. Documenting the early response in the United States, the author Randy Shilts (himself now dead from AIDS) observed in 1987 that there were 'endless stories' about the spread of the disease amongst heterosexuals: 'No hint that the disease might spread to straights, no matter how specious, was too small to put on page one.'

But the alarm was by no means confined to media sensationalism. During 1986, President Ronald Reagan's Surgeon-General, Dr Everett Koop, produced a far-sighted report that frankly addressed the broader public health issues arising from the epidemic. The report was important in that, coming from a member of an overtly right-wing, anti-gay administration, it warned against punitive and exclusionary measures against gay men with AIDS or HIV.

But Dr Koop also emphasised the broader public health implications of the epidemic. Because the risk was general, he advocated widespread use of condoms. And he urged that AIDS education for children should start at the earliest grade possible. The report outraged Reagan's far-right supporters who had originally supported Koop's appointment. But public health experts welcomed its wisdom in advocating protection for gay men and others living with HIV and AIDS, and in warning that a heterosexual epidemic was imminent.

But the heterosexual epidemic that so many feared and even expected in Western Europe and North America did not materialise. As HIV prevalence rates began to rise throughout central and southern Africa, as during the 1990s the high tide of the epidemic began washing inexorably southwards toward Africa's southern tip, the heterosexual infection rates in other parts of the world remained more or less constant. They stabilised at relatively low levels. In Europe and North America, AIDS even now is still largely confined to specific communities that are identified as being 'at risk' – men who have sex with men, injecting drug users, haemophiliacs, and their sexual partners.

Western European countries like the United Kingdom, the Netherlands, Spain and Norway have, according to UNAIDS figures, minimal disease prevalence – below 1 per cent – amongst adults of reproductive age. (In statisticians' language, 'reproductive age' generally refers to people between 15 and 49.) In Western Europe as a whole, HIV prevalence is a miniscule 0.3 per cent. In North America it is estimated to be much higher. Even so, prevalence there is 0.6 per cent, or just six people per thousand: a tiny fraction of that in many African countries.

In short, the heterosexual AIDS epidemic in these parts was and has remained a stunning non-event. After fervid coverage of the impending heterosexual AIDS threat in the mid-1980s, the London *Sunday Times* (reacting perhaps with self-induced discomfiture) resorted to advancing the views of dissident scientists, who denied that HIV was the cause of the catastrophic symptoms that were killing tens of thousands of gay men at the time. Rather than having a viral cause, the dissidents said, AIDS was the result of 'lifestyle choices' made by gay men (too much sex, too much partying, too many drugs). The symptoms conventional doctors ascribed to HIV disease they attributed to 'the long-term consumption of recreational drugs' and to the widespread use of drugs as sexual stimulants by homosexual men.

Given that with the onset of the epidemic most gay men instantly shrank away from all 'lifestyle choices' claimed to be the cause of AIDS, and that many who had indulged themselves most extravagantly in parties, drugs and sex remained totally unaffected, the theory was demonstrably ridiculous. As the death toll amongst gay men continued to mount, the dissident scientists fell back on the suggestion that what was killing the patients was AZT and other anti-retroviral drugs that doctors were wrong-headedly prescribing for AIDS. Certainly doctors erred in the late 1980s and early 1990s when they prescribed AZT and other antiretroviral drugs as single therapy. But that is not because the drugs, in the carefully controlled doses that were administered, were toxic to patients with AIDS. It was because in monotherapy each drug was ineffective – the virus found ways around it. It was only when AZT and other antiretroviral drugs were combined with at least two other drugs in the early to mid-1990s that their dramatic efficacy in suppressing the virus was discovered.

Yet a decade later, as we shall see, the 'AIDS drugs are toxic' theory had tragic life-and-death consequences in Africa when it attracted high political support.

The non-event of heterosexual HIV/AIDS is equally remarkable outside Europe and North America. Apart from sub-Saharan Africa, AIDS amongst heterosexuals just does not seem to have grown into the problem that once seemed to threaten. In Australia and New Zealand, HIV and AIDS affect less than one-tenth of one per cent of the population. Australasian health specialists are reasonably sure that all those who have HIV or AIDS are intravenous drug users or men who have sex with men. No wider outbreak has occurred or seems feasible. In the 1980s Australia from the outset implemented vigorous but rational and fair public health measures. These ensured that the epidemic remained confined within very narrow limits.

Also in South and South-East Asia and in East Asia and the Pacific, the prevalence remains low. Amongst young adults (15-49) it is for now still well below 1 per cent.

Professor William Makgoba, a South African university vice-chancellor and former head of the Medical Research Council, uses his speeches on AIDS to contrast the position in South Africa with that in Thailand. He does so by highlighting a particular figure – in 1990, the HIV prevalence rate in both South Africa and Thailand was 0.7 per cent (in other words, just above the present scope of infection amongst North Americans). A decade later, the rate in Thailand had stabilised at less than 2 per cent. At the end of 2001, UNAIDS estimated the HIV prevalence amongst Thais of reproductive age to be 1.8 per cent – disquietingly higher, of course, than in the United States or Western Europe, but still manageably low; and, more important, stable.

But in South Africa in the same period estimated HIV prevalence amongst young adults rocketed to near 20 per cent. Whereas AIDS amongst Thais was almost exclusively confined to communities defined as being 'at risk', in South Africa UNAIDS estimated that about one in five or six young adults – heterosexual adults – faced death from AIDS. In the first fifteen years of South Africa's epidemic, from 1982 to 1997, experts estimate that nearly 80 per cent of HIV transmission was heterosexual. Thirteen per cent was from mother to child ('MTCT'). One per cent was through infected blood supplies. And only 7 per cent was stated as being through men having sex with men. (Professor Makgoba however points out provocatively to audiences that African culture countenanced man-man sexual relations long before Europeans colonised the continent: I have heard animated cries of discomfited and amused recognition when audiences hear him pronounce the ancient sePedi word 'matanyola', signifying male/male sex: he asserts that the role of homosexual transmission of HIV in Africa is significantly under-recognised and understated.)

The difference between the epidemic in Africa and that in the rest of the world is pronounced and undeniable. As a mass problem, heterosexual AIDS at present seems just about confined to the African continent. Here, almost unimaginable levels of HIV are threatening the 'general' population. (In the discreet terminology epidemiologists use, this means non-gay, non-drug-injecting people.) In Swaziland, a landlocked kingdom wedged between South Africa and Mozambique, prevalence amongst young adults was estimated in 2003 at more than 38 per cent. In South Africa's western neighbour, Botswana, the estimate at that time was 37 per cent – a fractional decline from the previous year, when it was reportedly the highest in the world.

In 2003 the Ministry of Health and Social Welfare in Lesotho (a small mountain kingdom encircled by South Africa's Eastern Cape, KwaZulu-Natal and Free State provinces) conducted a survey of 2 666 women at six sentinel sites. The survey was 'anonymous unlinked'. This means that not only are the blood samples unnamed, but that there is no number, code, locality, clinic or doctor's name to link the blood sample to the donor. The survey revealed a median HIV prevalence of 28.5 per cent. This corresponded closely to the UNAIDS estimate for 2003 of 28.9 per cent amongst young adults. In Zimbabwe to the north, the estimated prevalence in 2003 was one-quarter of the young adult population. In Zambia, it was reckoned at 16.5 per cent. In Malawi, the 2002 estimate was lower. There, a mere 15 per cent of young adults – 'only' three out of every twenty – seemed to face death from AIDS.

Only a fool would say that no heterosexual epidemic can or will ever occur outside Africa. It is more prudent to say that a mass heterosexual epidemic has not yet manifested itself elsewhere. It could still happen. The proportion of women with AIDS or HIV in South and South-East Asia and in East Asia and the Pacific is troublingly high – between one-quarter and one-third of all AIDS or HIV cases. This is much higher than in North America or Western Europe. This implies that a heterosexual epidemic could yet develop. Wisely, public health officials are treating it exactly so. The same applies in China, where one-fifth of all humans live. Surveillance data are sketchy, but estimates are that nearly a million Chinese already have HIV or AIDS. And reported cases of HIV infection rose by more than two-thirds in the first half of 2001. To call the possibility of a widespread HIV epidemic amongst Chinese a 'spectre', as UNAIDS does, does not seem exaggerated.

In Eastern Europe, too, there are worrying signs that a more generalised epidemic could occur. Though prevalence there is still miniscule (less than 1 per cent), in the Russian Federation cases of HIV and AIDS are rising. And a rash of new cases amongst women suggests the disquieting possibility of a far greater spread of HIV than in Western Europe.

Yet with strong political commitment from top government leaders, and proper management at lower levels, even a nascent threat of HIV spread can be contained. That is the story of how Thailand has managed HIV over the last ten or fifteen years. And that story may derive support from the case of Cambodia.

So which way will an epidemic go? It is impossible to predict. Take

India. Since 1999 I have journeyed there three times (and, as I finalise these pages for typesetting, a fourth trip is planned for January 2005). My journeys have been with Australian High Court justice Michael Kirby, a hero of the early years of AIDS awareness, and still one of the clearest voices for rationality and justice in the epidemic. Kirby is a wonderful travelling companion, providing intensity, purpose and humour on what he calls our 'caravans' through India.

They have taken us to workshops, meetings and conferences with judges, parliamentarians and politicians in some of the subcontinent's most imposing and intriguing cities – Mumbai, Delhi, Ahmedabad, Surat, Bangalore, Cochin, Trivandrum. At each meeting our message is simple but unmistakable. Take early action. Do not be complacent. Avoid victimising people with AIDS or HIV and those at risk of acquiring it.

Kirby makes an insistent point about what he calls 'the AIDS paradox'. This is the insight that human rights and HIV containment go together. Sound reasons, rooted not only in respect for human dignity but in effective public health planning, demand a nondiscriminatory, human rights response to AIDS. Recognition of and respect for individual rights do not impede the prevention of HIV, he tells our audiences – they actually enhance containment, because they enable those infected or at risk of infection to come forward for testing, counselling, education and – where available – treatment.

With our hosts – the European Union-funded Lawyers Collective HIV/AIDS Unit in Mumbai – we urge the Indian authorities and judges to take early precautionary action to curtail the risk of a mass outbreak of HIV in India. We counsel rational, just and far-sighted measures in relation to Indians already living with HIV, who in some estimates are already said to number up to five million.

Our journeys have left ineradicable impressions of India's generosity and hospitality. And our meetings with cabinet ministers in Delhi, and with the chief ministers of some of India's states, as well as with legislators and with High Court and Supreme Court judges, have seemed well directed and productive. Yet after each of our 'caravans' I have battled with nagging doubts. A working journey through India can be hugely draining – every transport, every transfer, every stop an arduous effort. More than once – despite care in what I eat and drink – I have been felled by Western-unfriendly tummy bugs. So I end up asking myself: was the expense and the effort really warranted?

How likely is it that a mass-based epidemic in India really will eventuate? Will India's epidemic take the southern African form? Or will the current fear of a heterosexual epidemic prove to be merely an echo of the anxieties British politicians and public health planners fell prey to in the mid-1980s, an insubstantial phantasm that will take no firm shape or form? In ten years' time, if India's epidemic has the shape of Thailand's (low prevalence; infections confined largely to identified 'risk' groups) then surely our puny contribution to avoiding the eventuality – all the arrangements, preparations, flights, hotel bookings, meals, transport, early mornings, late nights, workshops, meetings, speeches, debates, persuasive energies (and occasionally attendant tummy rumbles) – would have been better directed elsewhere?

At present there seems to be little evidence that any generalised spread of HIV is taking place in India. One balmy night in early 2002, in the warm winter of India's south, after a long day addressing a packed gathering of lawyers and public health officials at the university in Trivandrum (or, to give the name of Kerala's capital its full Malayalam-language splendour, 'Thiruvananthapuram'), followed by a meeting with Kerala's chief minister, Mr AK Antony, and his entourage of officials, I expressed these doubts to our Indian hosts Anand Grover and Vivek Divan, as our hired eight-seater van transported Kirby and me back to our hotel in Kochi. The six-hour drive was bumpy and more than occasionally perilous. It matched the peaks and pitfalls of our conversation. 'Where is this huge Indian epidemic you have been warning us about repeatedly?' I demanded of our tour leader Anand, a great-hearted, gregarious man whose handsome charm, deep political convictions and legal polish have helped win court victories for India's poor and dispossessed.

Anand's indignant retort was bolstered by a passionate Vivek. The official figures are poorly kept and unreliable. They fail, he insisted, to reveal the current extent of HIV infections, still less the ambit of the potential crisis ahead. An epidemic of African proportions looms – or at least, he insists, it is folly to assume that it may not eventuate. A recent study by the University of California's AIDS Research Institute (ARI) at San Francisco gives Vivek's cautionary words credence. ARI emphasises that it is hard to be sure about the level of HIV infection in India, and that controversy continues to surround the exact figures.

India's government-created National AIDS Control Organisation (NACO) adds its cautious voice. It believes that AIDS is no longer affecting only 'high-risk' groups or urban populations, but is gradually spreading into rural areas and into what epidemiologists call 'the general population'. (When confronted, no epidemiologist will of course defend the suggestion implicit in this terminology that gay men are not part of 'the general population'.) In July 2003, NACO released new figures suggesting that the number of Indians with HIV or AIDS was between 3.8 and 4.5 million. Of these, nearly two-fifths are estimated to be women. As elsewhere in Asia, this is a worrying pointer to a potentially wide-spreading epidemic.

What is more, the ARI study emphasises, the low overall prevalence – less than half of one per cent of the total population of just over one billion – masks crucial differences between India's regions, states and subpopulations. That night on the road from Trivandrum, as blissfully haphazard oncoming traffic occasionally forced our driver to veer off the road, our debate proved inconclusive. I remained sceptical, pointing to the persisting and (I think) telling absence of clear data signalling an impending mass epidemic. And Anand and Vivek remained emphatic that the risk continued to be real.

So more 'caravans' I hope there will be. If India's epidemic does eventually match that of southern Africa, it will not be for want of plain-spoken warnings. But we may look back on India's preparations for a mass epidemic and find that – blessedly – it was as unlikely to eventuate as heterosexual AIDS in Western Europe and North America in the mid-1980s. Or in Thailand in the mid-1990s, just further down the map of the south Asian subcontinent, whose contained epidemic now furnishes Professor Makgoba with such a poignant contrast to our own predicament in Africa.

But perhaps – rather than worrying about the reasons for an African heterosexual epidemic – the issue can be conjured away. What if there is no heterosexual epidemic in Africa? What if, even in Africa, the spectral prophecy of a mass epidemic is unwarranted – perhaps an illusion – possibly even a phantasm deliberately figmented by activists and bureaucrats intent on exaggerating the epidemic for selfish career motives?

Some AIDS sceptics point out that there is no absolutely certain proof of the extent of HIV infection in Africa. Their argument stems from the acknowledged fact that figures predicting disease catastrophe in Africa are estimates – no more than the informed guesses of statisticians and medical experts. No one thinks of them as precise. It is difficult, for one thing, to make reliable projections from any 'sentinel' method of survey – this is the method that takes small samples of a population and projects its findings into the general population. In HIV prevalence studies, 'sentinel surveys' usually come from antenatal clinics, where women seek help during pregnancy. These are often poor women. Or the figures come from clinics that concentrate on treating sexually transmitted infections (STIs). Since the stigma of a sexually acquired disease drives those who have the money to seek help privately, such public clinics usually serve poorer, more disease-vulnerable populations.

So the surveys on which African figures are based establish the rate of HIV infection only amongst selected and relatively small groups. The epidemiologists then try to work out what HIV rates in these groups suggest about overall prevalence. But many factors might skew the results when projected onto a vast national canvas. For instance, if poor women attending antenatal clinics are more prone to HIV than other women, or if those seeking treatment for sexually transmitted infections are more likely to have HIV than the rest of the population, unadjusted projection would give grossly distorted results.

The statisticians acknowledge these problems. What is more, the UNAIDS figures (as I pointed out earlier) are generally for people in the 15-to-49 age group. Add the middle-aged, elderly and very young – all much less likely to have HIV than young adults in the prime of their sexual lives – and figures for a population as a whole could be very much lower. Indeed, problems of this sort have been shown to skew projections. In early 2004, a national prevalence study released in Kenya suggested that the UNAIDS figures for that country could be overstated by about one-quarter. At the end of 2001, UNAIDS estimated HIV prevalence in Kenya amongst young adults at about 15 per cent. By contrast, a household survey (in which researchers target selected homes, asking family members for saliva samples for HIV testing) showed that total national prevalence could in fact be under 7 per cent. The UNAIDS figures, adjusted for the whole population (as opposed to only sexually active young adults) would have come out at just over 9 per cent – a not insignificant two-percent difference.

In October 2004, the United Nations reported on a new survey released by Cameroon's health ministry. This indicated a drop in the number of adults living with HIV/AIDS. According to preliminary results of a survey conducted between October 2003 and August 2004, the national HIV prevalence rate is 5.5 per cent – much lower than an earlier estimate of 11.8 per cent. The new figure is less than half that extrapolated from the 2003 sentinel survey of pregnant women at antenatal clinics. The figure is, however, close to the UNAIDS figure of 6.9 per cent, which used calculations based on information from wider sources.

Does the debate about how precisely bad AIDS is in Africa matter? Surely whether it's ten or fifteen or thirty million Africans makes no difference?

The answer is that of course it makes a difference. Most obviously, the fewer people at risk of dying of AIDS, the better. So any reliable suggestion that the estimates may be overstated is good news. The figures matter also for another reason. How we think of a problem, the urgency and priority we accord it, depends in part on the size of the claim it makes upon our imagination. And the more people we think of as vulnerable to AIDS, the more our imagination is (or at least should be) engaged with it. So any exaggeration or misstatement in the UNAIDS figures should lead us to feel not just a sense of relief and reprieve. It should make us feel that we have been misled into undue alarm by an over-loud cry of 'wolf'. It is this justified resentment of misguided and irresponsible claims upon our sympathies that some AIDS sceptics have exploited in a recent controversy.

Yet are the conventional figures wrong in any sense that should affect the practical response to AIDS? How loud – and how false – has the cry about the extent of Africa's epidemic been? If the town watchboy thinks he sees an approaching pack of forty wolves, and only fifteen or twenty show up, should he not have cried wolf at all? Should the smaller number affect the town's watchfulness or its preparations – or its sense of debt to the boy's vigilance?

In practical terms, how much difference can it make that UNAIDS estimated that at the end of 2001 there were 28.5 million people in sub-Saharan Africa living with HIV/AIDS, if eventually it were shown that the true figure is in fact only fifteen or twenty million? Or some other proportion – perhaps three-quarters, or a quarter, of the UNAIDS estimate? Should it really affect anything we are currently doing or thinking (or should be doing or thinking) if there are only fifteen, or twenty, or twelve, or ten, or eight million Africans who risk dying of AIDS?

The answer is 'no'. By any calculations, Africa's AIDS epidemic is desperately under-resourced. On even the most conservative projections, too little is being done to care for those whom AIDS currently threatens. It is not as though the world is already doing enough for twenty or thirty million needy people with AIDS, efforts now wasted because the true figure is 'only' fifteen million. It is not doing enough even for the lowest conceivable estimates.

So even if the figures are half or less than the international projections, AIDS is still an international emergency that demands more, not less, drastic and immediate action. Nothing currently planned is inappropriate to an epidemic that might be only half or less the size of the worst UNAIDS predictions.

But the debate about statistics can cloak a deeper scepticism about AIDS. Some sceptics merely have reservations about the accuracy of the epidemiologists' forecasts. They do not doubt the brute fact of the epidemic. Others have exploited uncertainty about Africa's AIDS figures in pursuit of a darker purpose in the debate about AIDS. One writer has made a sensation about the accuracy of UNAIDS estimates, arguing that apparent over-estimates are not only 'grotesque' but sinister. He sees inflated figures as evidence of an 'AIDS lobby' that punts 'fanatical' certainties.

An article in the London *Spectator* – penned by Rian Malan, a talented South African writer with a penchant for self-spotlighting sensation – has suggested that there are 'breeds' of AIDS activists and journalists who sound 'hysterical', coming forth on World AIDS Day 'like loonies drawn by a full moon'. He has implied that UNAIDS, in concert with what he calls a 'massive alliance of pharmaceutical companies, NGOs, scientists and charities' is engaged in a conspiracy to overstate the figures – and to do so deliberately.

Positions on the statistics debate are a pointer to underlying stances on the epidemic itself. Those who question whether AIDS really raises acute moral issues for governments, corporations, international institutions and political leaders seize upon statistical fuzziness as a chance to downgrade the ranking the epidemic enjoys in people's minds. Those who go even further, and doubt that AIDS exists at all as a specific condition caused by a virus, magnify the issue even more. AIDS denialists have seized on the statistics controversy as an opportunity to propagate suspicion and mistrust against those who see a significant international response to AIDS as vital to the lives of millions of poor people in Africa and elsewhere.

But to see the debate in perspective we must ask an elementary question. Accept that the figures are uncertain. Accept that they may be overstated. But why on earth would anyone deliberately exaggerate the dangers AIDS poses to Africans and other people? There is one possible answer, and Malan's *Spectator* article was bold enough to give it credence. It is that an international entity that it calls 'the AIDS establishment' deliberately falsifies the risks AIDS poses to Africa because doing so will help it acquire money and power for itself. Malan goes so far as to endorse the suggestion that this 'establishment' is skilled at 'the manipulation of fear for advancement in terms of money and power'.

This is conspiracy thinking. It is the belief that events happen not for reasons that are apparent or that bear logical relation to their causes, but because powerful plotters acting for sinister, undisclosed and self-interested purposes secretly manipulate them. In this case, baldly stated, the conspiracy theory suggests that AIDS bureaucrats figment figures for power. It suggests, as the *Spectator* article did, that 'pharmaceutical companies, NGOs, scientists and charities' act in collusion with them for the same reasons.

If this strikes you as implausible, it is. It is on par with the hardy belief that a cabal of Jews secretly manipulates the international gold price for 'advancement in terms of money and power'. Unfortunately, both beliefs are still surprisingly widespread. The difference is that the anti-Semitic conspiracy theory would never be given precious space on the pages of the *Spectator*. The AIDS conspiracy theory is.

Why? Surely the theory is too bizarre for anyone to punt it? For many who have experienced first-hand the death and suffering that AIDS is wreaking in Africa, the theory is not only bizarre, but shocking and insulting. But if AIDS does not exist at all as a viral condition, then a conspiracy underlying the 'epidemic' is not so bizarre. In fact, if AIDS isn't caused by a virus, if it is a symptom not of a medical condition but of purely socio-environmental factors that lead to immune breakdown, if there is no need for AIDS drugs to save lives in Africa, then such thinking would be necessary and salutary. And if these facts are known (or should be known), then of course international AIDS bureaucrats, in alliance with 'pharmaceutical companies, NGOs, scientists and charities', must be exaggerating the AIDS statistics for sinister, misbegotten and selfish purposes.

If the science that claims to establish the existence of HIV, its causal link to AIDS, and the threat the virus poses to human life in Africa is distorted, unreliable and untruthful, then conspiracy thinking appears less extravagant. Then 'the AIDS establishment' must have sinister motives in overstating an epidemic that, if only truth could prevail, the world will see is not happening at all.

And this is the heart of the matter. In Africa, the collision of epidemiology with race and politics has led to bizarre deviations from rational debate on the causes of – and the possible treatments for – AIDS. The cost to the continent – in lives and in public truth – has been very high.

Conventional scientific and medical wisdom about AIDS involves three central propositions. First, it is an infectious agent that causes AIDS. A pathogen, which scientists named the human immunodeficiency virus, passes from one human to another, lodging in the bodily fabric of each. Over time it is the activity of this virus that causes the immune breakdown that eventually leads to death from AIDS. Second, the virus is transmitted from one human to another in a small number of well-established ways, the most important of which is sexual intercourse. Third, the catastrophic effects of HIV infection in its late stages can be prevented and even reversed by administering antiretroviral drugs that bring the activity of the virus that causes AIDS to a halt within the human body.

The vast majority of the world's scientists and medical doctors accept these premises as elementary: they do so because by every accepted criterion of scientific hypothesis and inference, the conventional approach to AIDS stands established. They therefore accept that AIDS is a virally caused, medically manageable condition that is mostly transmitted by sex. This view is supported by exhaustive clinical and laboratory evidence, and by overwhelming case studies – and by the first-hand experience of patients, doctors, families, friends and colleagues who have seen the effects of AIDS in North America, Europe and Africa.

This does not mean that current insights into the aetiology and epidemiology of AIDS are complete, exhaustive and beyond improvement. No scientific theory ever is. Knowledge advances slowly, incrementally, and as we learn more about ourselves and our world we will learn more about AIDS. There are still many intractable puzzles about the disease and the epidemic. Only more research and insight will resolve them.

But according to accepted precepts of scientific deduction, there is no doubt that the syndrome of opportunistic diseases that presented itself amongst the gay men of North America and Western Europe in the early 1980s, and that is now ravaging subcontinental Africa, is triggered by a viral, infectious condition.

That conventional wisdom is sombre. But it is also hopeful. It entails a further belief. That large-scale production and distribution and administration of antiretroviral drugs – under proper medical supervision, and in suitable socio-economic conditions – to the millions who without them would die must be the starting point of any rational, humane response to the epidemic.

But some contest these beliefs at their core – they dispute that AIDS is caused by a virus. So they contest the other premises with indignant and angry bitterness. They dispute that HIV is sexually transmitted. Some even consider that the suggestion that Africans in large numbers have acquired HIV infection through sex is a racial insult.

So the scientific and medically supported beliefs about AIDS remain only the 'conventional' wisdom on the disease. This is because the accepted approach is hotly, angrily, even desperately disputed by a small group of denialists. To the majority, who operate by the accepted canons of scientific inference, deduction and refutation, these researchers are intellectual and moral outcasts who discredit their own capacity for reason by defying the elementary premises of rational thinking and scientific inference.

But to their supporters, they are Galileo-like heroes, bravely defying blind orthodoxy in the name of truth.

In Africa, the issue is not merely intellectual or academic. Here the debate about the nature and causes of AIDS involves decisions that entail life and death – that exact lives and deaths in the many thousands. And differing positions on AIDS have cost many lives – perhaps as many as, or more than, some of the continent's other tragic but more obviously bloody encounters with death in the last few decades. This is because the dissidents' claims have attracted surprising support in Africa.

Why should the dissident views be attractive? And why should the conventional wisdom on AIDS be at all controversial? In an age in which medical science has made extraordinary advances, in which more diseases and disabling conditions can be medically treated and managed than at any stage in human history, in which we look to scientific explanations and rely on medical guidance, why should the aetiology of AIDS, vouched for by more laboratory, physiological, and epidemiological data than almost any other viral affliction, be at all suspect?

The beginning of this chapter gives the answer: race and sex. And the previous chapter gives the underlying clue: stigma.

If – however uncertain the figures, and however unreliable disease forecasting – a mass heterosexual epidemic of HIV and of AIDS deaths is taking place in central and southern Africa, if millions of Africans have HIV and are dying from AIDS (whether they be 28 million or ten or fourteen million), this leads to an overwhelming question: why Africa? What makes Africa – and particularly central Africa and the southern subcontinent – so different from the rest of the world?

Epidemiologists have been puzzling about this since the mid-1980s when it became clear that Africa's epidemic was more concentrated, more severe and more widespread than anywhere else in the world. Some think that poverty and the lack of healthcare facilities, particularly in treating sexually transmitted infections, explain the massive differences in HIV infection patterns between Africa and the rest of the world. But poverty and poor healthcare are not unique to Africa. Neither India nor Thailand have significantly better health facilities than are available to most Africans. And the poverty-stricken conditions in which hundreds of millions of Asians live are by no means dissimilar to those in Africa.

Others specialists cite Africa's wars, dislocation, mobile populations and migratory workers. These features, again, have contributed considerably to the spread of HIV. But they are not unique to Africa, nor even unique to the parts of Africa where the epidemic has hit hardest. West Africa has been plagued by many armed conflicts and by dislocation and population shifts – yet currently HIV infection there is still significantly lower than in central and southern Africa. According to UNAIDS the countries with the highest prevalence in West Africa currently are war-torn Liberia, with an adult prevalence of 5.9 per cent, Nigeria with 5.4 per cent, and Togo, with 4.1 per cent. These are appreciably lower than the infection rates in most southern African countries. In most other West African countries (Senegal: 0.5 per cent; Ghana: 3.1 per cent; Guinea: 3.2 per cent; Gambia: 1.2 per cent), the disparity is even greater.

What then can the reason be? For some, this is the Big Question in the African debate about AIDS. And the range of possible answers has at times bedevilled rational thinking about the epidemic. This is because one obvious possibility is sexual behaviour. Perhaps, some think, the epidemic in central and southern Africa is different from elsewhere because people in central and southern Africa have sex differently or more often or with more partners. More than 90 per cent of HIV transmissions are through sexual intercourse. So surely, they argue, differences in disease rates must reflect differences in sexual behaviour?

Amongst gay men, where the disease first manifested itself in the early 1980s, it is accepted that sex, sex with more partners, almost certainly sex with too many partners, led to the horrific toll the disease took on the gay communities of San Francisco and London and New York. Randy Shilts recalled with aching poignancy how in the late 1970s sex for gay men 'was part and parcel of political liberation'. Having a great deal of sex with different partners, freely, was an expression of political freedom. Gay leaders and spokesmen, and the doctors and scientists serving the gay community, made no bones about naming the cause of transmission – and telling gay men to change their sexual habits. The most intensely debated issue in the 1980s was sex and sexual behaviour and how to react to the threat of death spread by it.

But – crucially – the issue was not only sex and how much of it gay men were having with too many partners. It was also physiology – gay men are peculiarly susceptible to HIV transmission during sex. For distinct bodily reasons (the permeability and fragility of the mucosal rectal lining), anal intercourse makes the receptive partner very much more vulnerable to HIV transmission than heterosexual intercourse.

So what about sexual conduct in Africa? UNAIDS emphasises the significant variations between cultures, age groups, genders and socioeconomic classes in Africa. Then quietly but unmistakably it adds, 'sexual behaviour is the most important factor influencing the spread of HIV in Africa'. So is that it? Sex is 'the most important factor'. An epidemic of death on the world's 'dark continent', enmeshed with sex, and fuelled by the distinctive sexual habits and behaviour of the inhabitants of central and southern Africa? It is the laden implications of this suggestion that has skewed rational discussion of the epidemic.

Despite huge strides in sexual openness and public discussion, sexual behaviour and cultural differences remain a fraught topic. This is rightly so. Sex is the most intimate physical act two people can perform together. Rightly, it generally takes place in private, between consenting adults. Seclusion may be necessary to give us a haven for expression and release of inmost feelings that do not easily countenance daylight. I suggested in Chapter Two that a large part of the stigma that attaches to HIV derives from the fact that it is mostly sexually transmitted. This in turn stems from the vestigial sense of shame we seem to feel when our moments of sexual connection and sexual release are marked by or evidenced in a sexually acquired infection or illness.

It is even more fraught to raise these questions in relation to an epidemic in Africa. White colonialists have a long and shameful history of salacious preoccupation with black sexual behaviour. Shakespeare and Mozart reflect that history, although their treatment is moderated with subtlety and complexity. Other Western violations of Africans and their culture have been entirely lacking in subtlety. A San woman, named Saartjie Baartman, was transported to Europe in 1810 as 'the black Venus' or 'the Hottentot Venus'. She was paraded as an exemplar of prodigious black sexual capacities because of the supposed size of her genitals. Not even in death was her body accorded dignity: it was dismembered and continued to be displayed until the late twentieth century in the Musee de l'Homme in Paris. Her remains were returned to South Africa only in May 2002 after a resolution of the French Parliament permitted their repatriation, and were laid to rest in a moving ceremony on the banks of the Gamtoos River near her birthplace at Hankey in the Eastern Cape in August 2002.

White stereotyping of black sexuality and sexual conduct continues into the 21st century. It is scarcely surprising that discussion of differential disease patterns in AIDS can verge on the explosive. Nor is it wholly surprising that at least some in Africa allege that the conventional approach to HIV entails a damning judgment on Africans' sexual behaviour. They see in this a consolidation of hundreds of years of prurient Western preoccupation with African sexuality and sexual behaviour.

This has led to a distinctive African form of AIDS denialism. This is premised, like the convictions of the denialists who exploit the statistics issue, on a belief in conspiracy. But in Africa it has racial overtones: the conspiracy is racially inspired. The African AIDS deniers depict the facts about AIDS as the product of a grotesque racist conspiracy of untruth and deception by corporations, doctors, scientists and healthcare workers – designed to humiliate and exploit Africans because they are black.

In April 2002 a disturbing document was distributed within the structures of the African National Congress, the ruling party in South Africa. It took the form of a long (114-page) treatise on AIDS and its causes. Of uncertain authorship, it was preoccupied with concerns about the toxicity of the drugs conventional doctors insisted Africa needed to prevent millions of AIDS deaths. It expressed the view that a syndicate of white Western interests – an 'omnipotent apparatus' – was engaged in 'a massive political-commercial campaign to promote antiretroviral drugs'. Through this campaign the 'apparatus' sought to degrade, exploit and eventually by the administration of toxic antiretroviral medicines, kill Africans.

The author or authors seem to believe that the conventional approach to AIDS imputes inordinate sexual over-exertions to Africans in those countries where the epidemic has reached mass proportions:

'Yes, we are sex-crazy! Yes, we are diseased! Yes, we spread the deadly HI Virus through our uncontrolled heterosexual sex! In this regard, yes, we are different from the US and Western Europe! Yes, we, the men, abuse women and the girl-child with gay abandon! Yes, among us rape is endemic because of our culture! Yes, we do believe that sleeping with young virgins will cure us of AIDS! Yes, as a result of all this, we are threatened with destruction by the HIV/AIDS pandemic! Yes, what we need, and cannot afford because we are poor, are condoms and antiretroviral drugs! Help!'

The irony may be painfully heavy-handed. But the message is clear: belief in the conventional predicates of epidemiology and disease management as they apply to AIDS in Africa is racist because it proceeds from the premise that HIV is mostly sexually transmitted.

The document was never officially repudiated by the ANC. Some of its main themes seemed to have the support of President Mbeki. In a speech six months earlier to a university audience at Fort Hare in the Eastern Cape, he made a heartfelt call for new thinking about race and personhood – a 'revolution in the minds not only of Africans but of all humanity, so that Africa could overcome the legacy of centuries of slavery and colonialism'. But he also appeared to castigate AIDS activists for harping on the mounting crisis of disease and death in South Africa. Their conduct, he seemed to imply, proceeded from racist hypotheses about Africans, wrongly presented as facts:

'Thus does it come about that some who call themselves our leaders join a cacophony of voices that demand that we produce statistics that will show that, indeed, we belong to the most criminal element in our country. And thus does it happen that others who consider themselves to be our leaders take to the streets carrying their placards, to demand that because we are germ carriers, and human beings of a lower order that cannot subject its passions to reason, we must perforce adopt strange opinions, to save a depraved and diseased people from perishing from self-inflicted disease . . . Convinced that we are but natural-born, promiscuous carriers of germs, unique in the world, they proclaim that our continent is doomed to an inevitable mortal end because of our unconquerable devotion to the sin of lust.'

Against this background, the distribution of the ANC document – and suggestions that its provenance commanded high approval – cast a sombre shadow over the AIDS debate in South Africa. Within influential governmental circles, for agonising months, eventually years, public debate about AIDS, its treatment and its causes seemed to come to a virtual dead stop. Support for the facts about HIV transmission and AIDS treatments seemed a heresy to which no government minister would adhere.

But does the conventional approach to AIDS stigmatise Africans as sex-mad fiends? I don't think so. Not only is it wrong to moralise scientific explanation, but science does not necessarily entail what the African AIDS dissidents impute to it.

Inevitably, I'm asked my opinion at policy and educational and awareness meetings. I disclaim expertise, emphasising my obvious limitations. I am not a virologist, not a demographer, not a sociologist, not an epidemiologist, not even – except to the extent that legal practice and judicial duties necessitate it – a student of human character. But I give my view. Not to do so would be evasive. Anyhow it seems obvious to me. Africans in our subcontinent do not behave so differently from Europeans or North Americans or Indians or Cambodians or people in Thailand that this can explain our distinctive mass epidemic.

I have never accepted the solely sexual explanation of Africa's differential disease pattern. If it suggests that the people of central and southern Africa have so much more intercourse, so differently, or with so many more partners, than people elsewhere in the world, and that this is why so far they alone have experienced a mass heterosexual epidemic of HIV, I do not believe it.

What is it then? I'm not sure. At a dinner in Sandton, Johannesburg, in the mid-1990s, Professor Luc Montagnier of Paris's Pasteur Institute, who a decade earlier first isolated the virus that causes AIDS, voiced the opinion across the table that there may be distinctive genetic features that render some Africans more vulnerable to HIV transmission than people elsewhere. Enter physiology and genetics as explanations, then, rather than just behaviour. And add the environment. And add social causes such as poverty, insufficient healthcare, and commercially or politically forced migrancy.

To me these causes, in various possible combinations, seem to offer a far more plausible account than any solely behavioural explanation for the mass viral transmission in Africa. Perhaps the human body's subtle genetic variations create pathways in some people that allow the virus to enter more readily than in others. Perhaps this, in combination with the fact that many Africans have previous or present exposure to other disease-causing pathogens, and perilously fewer healthcare facilities than most other people, and have been forced by war and economic need into many pathogen-spreading patterns of migrancy, explains our special subcontinental vulnerability to infection by HIV and AIDS sickness.

During a research fellowship I held in the last months of 2003 at All Souls, one of Oxford's most beautiful and ancient colleges, a mediaeval historian made an intriguing observation to me that bolstered my scepticism about the suggestion that sexual behaviour alone could explain the epidemic's African concentration. Intrigued by what I had told him of the seemingly inexplicable disease patterns of HIV, he asked whether I knew that the great bubonic plague of the mid-1300s had left certain parts of Europe virtually untouched? The Low Countries (the Netherlands and present-day Belgium) went almost unscathed, he explained, and the same applied to Portugal and to large areas of Poland.

Historians and disease specialists still debate what particular pathogen caused the mid-fourteenth century plague, and those that followed it in later centuries. They are not unanimous that it was what we call 'plague' today – that is, rodent-borne fleas infecting humans with a pathogen. But whatever it was, the destruction and devastation the disease wrought in its first manifestation seemed to leave some parts of Europe relatively untouched. Historical accounts are clear that while the Mediterranean countries were hardest hit, with England and Scandinavia also suffering huge population losses, Poland and the Low Countries were largely unscathed.

Why was this? No one knows. Mediaeval moralists and behaviourists undoubtedly expounded plausible-seeming explanations – that the people of the less-affected areas were more holy, more religious, more observant, less sinful. Perhaps they even proclaimed that the persons in the less-affected areas had less sinful sex than those where the plague hit hardest. We rightly look back on such explanations with indulgent condescension. Whatever the reason for the mysterious and as yet unexplained epidemiological pattern of the great plague, we know that it lies in pathogen, host and environment. It is not to do with sin or sex, and stigmatising the people who suffered is not only far-fetched but repugnant.

Yet similar undue moralism, and similar unscientific re-stigmatising theories, still plague the epidemiology of AIDS.

The fact is that we don't really know enough about how epidemics spread, nor about how differences between humans and the social and environmental settings in which they live make them more vulnerable to infection and to the onset of disease. We simply don't know enough about how microbes react to different human populations in different social settings. Perhaps this is an area where science still lacks solutions for the questions that the fourteenth century moralists tried to answer.

This is not to say that sexual conduct is unimportant. It is important. I have heard African women charge that they cannot negotiate sex freely on their own terms. Others report that they feel subordinated by men who claim an entitlement to have sex when they want to do so. Besides, sex and patterns of sexual behaviour obviously contribute to the growth of the epidemic in Africa. If all sexual intercourse throughout Africa suddenly stopped, the spread of HIV would stop – at least in nineteen out of twenty cases. So the focus on sex and sexual behaviour is unavoidable and necessary.

But Africans' susceptibility to HIV infection is not a judgment on their sexual conduct. Counter-scientific dissidence is misdirected, and unnecessary. It is also fatally damaging – of debate, and solutions. Africans may have sex just about the same or as often as people elsewhere, or with as many sequential partners as elsewhere, yet still find themselves more vulnerable to infection because of physiological and social conditions peculiar to the continent and the subcontinent.

And even if heterosexual Africans did behave differently in their frequency of sexual intercourse and their number of partners, why should that earn condemnation? The supposition is that frequency of sexual intercourse or variety of partners is in itself demeaning, revealing, shaming, degrading. Is it? We are back to self-stigma – internalised stigma – and its destructive, self-damaging effects. The combination of racial politics and self-stigma has cost us much time, and many lives, in Africa.

4 | The tragedy of AIDS denialism in South Africa

In late 1999, South Africa was estimated to have the highest number of people living with HIV/AIDS in the world – between four and five million, or 10 per cent of the entire population. A large proportion of those infected with HIV were already falling sick with AIDS, and dying. The epidemic was every day becoming more and more visible, its deadly reaping palpable in almost every family, workplace, township, farm, suburb, church and organisation.

Yet at this very time the country also entered a three-year nightmare period during which the cause-and-effect link between HIV and AIDS was officially questioned. This was no abstract, academic debate, conducted in scholarly journals and university seminar rooms. It emanated from the inner sanctum of governmental power in the country, and its domain was the entire spectrum of constructive political response to the AIDS epidemic.

Nor was the debate of theoretical import only. Its real consequence was life affecting – and all too desperately immediate. The significance of the doubt cast on HIV's causative role in AIDS was the fundamentally practical question of whether AIDS could be treated medically. If AIDS was merely a physical manifestation of environmental factors that cumulatively degrade human health – such as poverty and malnutrition and poor healthcare – then there would be no point in administering potentially toxic antiretroviral medications to those suffering its symptoms. On the contrary: in that case the drugs would just exacerbate the severe physiological malaise they were intended to arrest.

That was what was at issue when President Mbeki, who had taken office in succession to President Mandela as the country's second democratic president in mid-1999, rose to address Parliament on Thursday 28 October. In his speech he revealed his concern about the toxicity of the antiretroviral drug AZT. There was, he said, 'a large volume of scientific evidence alleging that, amongst other things, the toxicity of this drug is such that it is in fact a danger to health'.

It soon became clear that the president had become privy to the views propounded by dissident medical and social scientists who denied that HIV is the cause of AIDS. One of their central propositions is that the hundreds of thousands of deaths among gay men in Western Europe and North America in the 1980s and early 1990s, which medical science ascribes to a viral condition triggering immune collapse, were not in fact caused by the 'human immunodeficiency virus' at all. What caused them, the dissidents say, were first the 'lifestyle choices' wrongly made by affluent gay men (partying, drugs, too much sex) – and then the antiretroviral medications their doctors, acting in hideous folly and error, prescribed for their already-damaged immune systems.

The AIDS dissidents' dogma takes many forms. Some claim that HIV does not exist as a virus at all. Others assert that such a virus, if it exists at all, has never been isolated. Some urge that HIV does not exist as an infectious condition. Yet others assert that tests for HIV or its antibodies are wildly misleading and unreliable. They unite in claiming that, if it does exist at all, HIV has not been shown to be the cause of AIDS.

What we accept as 'scientific truth' – that light reaches our night skies from long-gone planets that encircled far-distant solar systems millions of years ago, that dinosaurs once roamed the earth, that those occupying the White House in Washington DC are not mutant aliens – is based on methods of scientific inquiry and evaluation that sift conjecture from theory from hypothesis from fact. No knowledge is totally certain. Nor is it ever fixed. Present postulates of physical science and chemistry may all be incorrect: but they will be superseded as scientific knowledge only when a more plausible theory, one that better fits all the available evidence, is propounded, as Einsteinian physics replaced that of Newton.

It was by honouring just these postulates of scientifically established inquiry and truth that Galileo Galilei asserted that the earth's solar system is heliocentric; and in dissidence from the same scientific postulates that the dogmatists of the church insisted that the earth, after all, was the centre of the universe.

By present-day methods of scientific experimentation, inquiry and evaluation of knowledge, it is abundantly established that a virus (which scientists have named for its effects on the human immune system) exists. It is also clear that its presence in the blood can be ascertained with great sensitivity and specificity. The virus is present in the overwhelming majority of cases of those persons, in Western Europe, North America and Africa, whose immune systems show the signs of disintegration that clinicians have called 'AIDS'. The workings of the virus – how it enters the cellular formations of the human immune system and destroys it – have been minutely and exhaustively and intricately documented and reported in laboratory, clinic and field.

It is on the basis of an overwhelming mass of clinical, scientific and experimental evidence, backed by field observations of many hundreds of healthcare personnel, that scientists and doctors say with relative certainty – subject to the revision of the postulates of human knowledge and understanding itself – that there is an epidemic of virally borne immune destruction plaguing much of central and southern Africa.

In the face of this very considerable body of evidence not only that HIV exists, but that it causes AIDS, and that it is devastating central and southern Africa, the denialists assert that the claim that AIDS is caused by a sexually transmitted virus is merely a 'hypothesis' – a hypothesis, they claim, that is not only unproven but irresponsible. They say that the statement that there is a microbial epidemic in Africa is merely an 'impression'. What is seen as a viral epidemic is really only the effect of 'non-contagious risk factors that are limited to certain sub-sets of the African population'. The millions of deaths – and the many tens of millions of expected deaths – attributed to AIDS they characterise as 'a minor fraction of conventional mortality under a new name'.

The words I have quoted are those of Professor Peter Duesberg, a California scientist whose thinking and writing has provided the platform for many of the AIDS denialists' claims over the last twenty years. But Duesberg's contentions and those of his adherents raise an important question. Why – if AIDS is but a mistaken 'impression' – would conventional medical science propound such a stunning falsehood? The denialists' answer is that many scientists are fools, trapped in dogmatic error. Others follow the herd, too unimaginative to think freely, innovatively and challengingly.

But all too many of them also have a baser motive. Their answer echoes that of the *Spectator* writer Rian Malan, whom I mentioned in Chapter Three. He saw a sinister profit-grasping motive behind over-stated AIDS figures. According to Duesberg, the 'deceptive AIDS propaganda' alleging the existence of a microbial AIDS epidemic in Africa has been 'introduced and inspired by new American biotechnology', one that – at least in the case of HIV testing – 'provides job security' for virologists and doctors, 'without ever producing any public health benefits'.

It was these views that President Mbeki pondered in late 1999 and early 2000. In March his spokesman Parks Mankahlana (who died a few months later, tragically young, from causes reported to be AIDS-related) announced that the president was to convene an international panel of experts to resolve questions about AIDS. The questions included 'whether there is this thing called AIDS, what it is, whether HIV leads to AIDS, whether there is something called HIV'.

In a letter to President Bill Clinton and other Western leaders in April 2000, President Mbeki pointed to the differences between the largely homosexual epidemic in Western countries and the overwhelmingly heterosexual manifestation of the epidemic in Africa. Consequently, he asserted, 'a simple superimposition of Western experience on African reality' would be not only 'absurd and illogical' – it would be a 'criminal betrayal of our responsibility to our own people'.

Critics of his AIDS review panel, he wrote, were engaged in an 'orchestrated campaign of condemnation'. Their suggestion that he should have no truck with dissident scientists because they were 'dangerous and discredited' worried him: 'At an earlier period in human history, these [dissident scientists] would be heretics that would be burnt at the stake.'

In a later exchange with a political opponent, opposition leader Tony Leon, he described claims about 'the African and Haitian origins of HIV' as 'wild and insulting'.

Soon after, Professor William Makgoba, one of the continent's most prominent medical research scientists, contributed an invited editorial to a leading scientific magazine. He charged that 'South Africa is rapidly becoming a fertile ground for the types of pseudoscience often embraced by politicians'. He damned as an absurd form of national denial what he called 'the politically motivated suggestion, in the absence of scientific evidence, that malnutrition and poverty cause AIDS in Africa'. He warned:

'The current political and scientific furore in South Africa, fuelled largely by the dissidents' theories on HIV/AIDS and the seeming support of Mr Mbeki, has much broader implications for South Africa and South Africans than some are prepared to admit. The current controversy is undermining the constructive public health messages this government has put in place. It is sending mixed messages to all those who have dedicated themselves to the alleviation and eradication of this epidemic and is having a negative impact on the morale of affected patients and families. The undermining of scientists and the scientific method is especially dangerous in a developing country still in the process of establishing a strong scientific research base. Furthermore, it may erode investor confidence in our country, with dire economic consequences. We present South Africans cannot afford to make any more mistakes lest history judges us to have collaborated in one of the greatest crimes of our time.'

Professor Makgoba's outspoken plea for rationality and logic in the AIDS debate has been bravely echoed, within South Africa, by distinguished leaders such as Archbishop Desmond Tutu, his successor Archbishop Njongonkulu Ndungane and Dr Mamphela Ramphele. Leading writers, journalists and intellectuals such as Justice Malala, Mondli Makhanya, Barney Mthombothi, Jovial Rantao, Ferial Haffajee, Khathu Mamaila, Pregs Govender, Prof Sipho Seepe and Dr Xolela Mangcu have spoken, in different ways, but to the same effect. Trade union leaders such as Willie Madisha and Zwelinzima Vavi and, within the medical field, Dr Olive Shisana and Dr Kgositsile Letlape, have amongst others been unflinching in their calls for truth. If all the names I mention are of black writers and intellectuals and leaders, it is because in a debate that took on such intense racial loading, their courage was particularly expressive.

As the world's AIDS specialists and workers prepared for the first international AIDS conference to be held within Africa, large numbers of distinguished scientists gave their support to Professor Makgoba's alarm call. In response to the establishment of the Presidential AIDS Advisory Panel, more than 5 000 physicians and scientists from 82 countries – all specialising in HIV/AIDS – signed the 'Durban Declaration of July 2000'. In it, they affirmed that the evidence that HIV causes AIDS is 'clear-cut, exhaustive and unambiguous'. It is supported, they said, by 'compelling data'. And it 'meets the highest standards of science'.

In opening the international AIDS conference in Durban in 2000, shortly before eleven-year-old Nkosi Johnson, himself sick with AIDS, spoke, the president seemed to chide these scientists, as well as conference-goers, for accepting HIV as the sole or even main causative factor in AIDS: 'The world's biggest killer and the greatest cause of ill health and suffering across the globe, including South Africa, is extreme poverty,' he said. He added: 'As I listened and heard the whole story about our own country, it seemed to me that we could not blame everything on a single virus.'

The president left immediately after his speech. He did not hear Nkosi's brave and moving plea for humane and inclusive action to deal with the epidemic and to mitigate its effects on those with HIV and AIDS.

Months before, in late 1999, the conference organisers had invited me to dedicate the keynote address at the opening session of the conference to the memory of Professor Jonathan Mann. Mann was the first head of the World Health Organisation's Global Programme on AIDS. His inspiring vision ensured that human rights norms were at the outset incorporated – for both humane and sensibly practical reasons – into public health approaches to the AIDS epidemic. He died tragically and prematurely when his Swissair flight crashed into the ocean off the eastern coast of the United States in September 1998.

When I accepted the organisers' invitation to honour Mann, I did not dream that the conference would occur against a tense and bitter backdrop of dissent about the usefulness of its taking place at all. For if the viral approach to AIDS was mistaken, then the gathering was of course a mightily mistaken waste of time and effort.

In honouring Mann's contribution to human rights norms in public health, I decided that my main target of attack had to be the close-fisted patents policies of the drug companies. Their products (which were regarded as the accepted approach to treatment) had dramatically curtailed death and serious illness from AIDS in the Western world. But in Africa – where the ravages of AIDS were most severely felt – those drugs were simply unavailable to the vast majority of those at risk of death.

I was an exception – one privileged by relative affluence to be alive. This I decided should be the main focus of my keynote. The drugs, I pointed out to nearly 14 000 delegates at the opening session on a balmy Durban winter's morning, were not miraculous: but in their physiological and social consequences they come very close to being miraculous.

'But this near-miracle has not touched the lives of most of those who most desperately need it. For Africans and others in resource-poor countries with AIDS and HIV, these drugs are out of reach. For them, the implications of the epidemic remain as fearsome as ever. In their lives, the prospect of debility and death, and the effects of discrimination and societal prejudice, loom as huge as they did for the gay men of North America and Western Europe a decade and a half ago.

'This is not because the drugs are prohibitively expensive to produce. They are not. Recent experience in India, Thailand and Brazil has shown that most of the critical drugs can be produced at a cost that puts them realistically within reach of the resource-poor world.'

The primary reason the drugs were inaccessible in the developing world was, I pointed out, the drug prices imposed by the manufacturers – which made the drugs unaffordably expensive; and the international patent and trade regime that choked off any large-scale attempt to produce and market the drugs at affordable levels. The divide between rich and poor, I said, threatened to swallow up 25 million lives in Africa:

'I speak of the gap not as an observer or as a commentator, but with intimate personal knowledge. I am an African. I am living with AIDS. I therefore count as one amongst the forbidding statistics of AIDS in Africa. I form part of nearly five million South Africans who have the virus. I speak also of the dread effects of AIDS not as an onlooker. Nearly three years ago, more than twelve years after I became infected, I fell severely ill with the symptomatic effects of HIV. Fortunately for me, I had access to good medical care. My doctor first treated the opportunistic infections that were making me feel sick unto death. Then he started me on combination therapy. Since then, with relatively minor adjustments, I have been privileged to lead a vigorous, healthy, and productive life. I am able to do so because, twice a day, I take two tablets . . . I can take these tablets because, on the salary of a judge, I am able to afford their cost.

'If, without combination therapy, the mean survival time for a healthy male in his mid-forties after onset of full AIDS is 30 to 36 months, I should be dead by about now. Instead, I am more healthy, more vigorous, more energetic, and more full of purposeful joy than at any time in my life.'

Some in the audience began to applaud joyfully at this point. But the point was not my feelings of wellbeing. I held up a cautionary hand:

'I exist as a living embodiment of the iniquity of drug availability and access in Africa. This is not because, in an epidemic in which the heaviest burden of infection and disease are borne by women, I am male; nor because, on a continent in which the vectors of infection have overwhelmingly been heterosexual, I am proudly gay; nor even because, in a history fraught with racial injustice, I was born white.

'My presence here embodies the injustices of AIDS in Africa because, on a continent in which 290 million Africans survive on less than one US dollar a day, I can afford monthly medication costs of about US $400 per month. Amidst the poverty of Africa, I stand before you because I am able to purchase health and vigour. I am here because I can afford to pay for life itself.

'To me this seems an iniquity of very considerable proportions – that, simply because of relative affluence, I should be living when others have died; that I should remain fit and healthy when illness and death beset millions of others.'

I went on to urge conference-goers to confront the moral challenge that drug access for poor people with AIDS posed to all of us:

'Moral dilemmas are all too easy to analyse in retrospect. It is often a source of puzzled reflection how ordinary Germans could have tolerated the moral iniquity that was Nazism; or how white South Africans could have countenanced the evils that apartheid inflicted, to their benefit, on the majority of their fellows.

'Yet the position of persons living with AIDS or HIV in Africa and other resource-poor countries poses a comparable moral dilemma for the developed world today. The inequities of drug access, pricing and distribution mirror the inequities of a world trade system that weighs the poor with debt while privileging the wealthy with inexpensive raw materials and labour.

'Those of us who live affluent lives, well-attended by medical care and treatment, should not ask how Germans or white South Africans could tolerate living in proximity to moral evil. We do so ourselves today, in proximity to the impending illness and death of many millions of people with AIDS. This will happen, unless we change the present. It will happen because available treatments are denied to those who need them for the sake of aggregating corporate wealth for shareholders who by African standards are already unimaginably affluent. That cannot be right, and it cannot be allowed to happen.

'No more than Germans in the Nazi era, nor more than white South Africans during apartheid, can we at this conference say that we bear no responsibility for more than thirty million people in resource-poor countries who face death from AIDS unless medical care and treatment is made accessible and available to them. The world has become a single sphere, in which communication, finance, trade and travel occur within a single entity. How we live our lives affects how others live theirs. We cannot wall off the plight of those whose lives are proximate to our own.'

The conference started the day after Zackie Achmat and the Treatment Action Campaign, joined by Anglican Archbishop Njongonkulu Ndungane, led a huge march to precede President Mbeki's official opening address. The marchers were demanding access to drugs.

Many consider that the challenge the TAC's activists directed to the Durban AIDS conference furnished the turning point in providing real progress to that goal.

But unfortunately those committed to saving lives through radical treatment-based interventions did not yet enjoy the support of the South African government. At the opening session the morning after the march, I felt compelled to speak also about the prevarication and dilatoriness of my own government's approach to AIDS:

'In my own country, a government that in its commitment to human rights and democracy has been a shining example to Africa and the world has at almost every conceivable turn mismanaged the epidemic. So grievous has governmental ineptitude been that South Africa has since 1998 had the fastest-growing HIV epidemic in the world. It currently has one of the world's highest prevalences . . . There has been a cacophony of task groups, workshops, committees, councils, policies, drafts, proposals, statements, pledges. But all have thus far signified piteously little.

'A basic and affordable measure would be a national programme to limit mother-to-child transmission of HIV through administration of short courses of antiretroviral medication. Research has shown this will be cost-effective in South Africa. Such a programme, if implemented, would have signalled our government's appreciation of the larger problem, and its resolve to address it. To the millions of South Africans living with HIV, it would have created a ray of light. It would have promised the possibility of increasingly constructive interventions for all with HIV, including enhanced access to drug therapies.

'To our shame, our country has not yet come so far as even to commit itself to implementing such a programme. The result, every month, is that 5 000 babies are born, unnecessarily and avoidably, with HIV. Their lives involve preventable infections, preventable suffering, preventable deaths. And if none of that is persuasive, then from the point of view of the nation's economic self-interest, their HIV infections entail preventable expense. Yet we have done nothing.'

Lastly, there was the fraught and painful subject of President Mbeki's engagement with the AIDS denialists. Earlier in the week, press speculation had reflected misguided hope that in opening the conference he would dispel the anxiety created by the effusion of dissident doctrines into the AIDS debate in South Africa, and instead unveil a programme to curb perinatal transmission of HIV. Some even believed that he would take the opportunity to renounce the confusion and uncertainty his AIDS review panel had caused.

Bitter disappointment followed his opening address. As someone living myself with AIDS, whose life had been saved by access to the new drugs, I felt I could not remain silent. Over breakfast at the Royal Hotel shortly before the conference was due to get down to business with its opening session at nine o'clock, I penned a careful addition to my prepared speech:

'In our national struggle to come to grips with the epidemic, perhaps the most intractably puzzling episode has been our president's flirtation with those who in the face of all reason and evidence have sought to dispute the aetiology of AIDS. This has shaken almost everyone responsible for engaging the epidemic. It has created an air of unbelief amongst scientists, confusion among those at risk of HIV, and consternation amongst AIDS workers.

'To my regret, I cannot believe that President Mbeki's speech at the official opening of this conference last night has done enough to counter these adverse conditions. I personally yearned for an unequivocal assertion from our president that HIV is a virally specific condition that is sexually transmitted, which if uncontained precipitates debility and death, but for which antiretroviral treatments now exist that can effectively and affordably be applied. To my grief, his speech was bereft of this.'

I then quoted one of Africa's foremost intellectuals, Dr Mamphela Ramphele, a former university head who has since become a leading World Bank executive. She described the official sanction given to scepticism about the cause of AIDS as 'irresponsibility that borders on criminality'. 'If this aberrant and distressing interlude has delayed the implementation of life-saving measures to halt the spread of HIV and to curtail its effects,' I said, 'then history will not judge this comment excessive.'

The inauguration of President Mbeki's AIDS Advisory Panel in 2000 initiated three years of tragic confusion in South African governmental approaches to AIDS. The consequences were severe. AIDS deaths mounted while government prevaricated on introducing mass access to antiretroviral medications. The doubt cast on the viral aetiology of AIDS was a massive setback also for prevention and education efforts. Public education about self-protection and the necessity for behaviour change is central to successful AIDS strategies. AIDS educators reported new difficulty in advancing safer-sex measures. On radio talk shows men openly stated that if HIV did not cause AIDS then it was pointless to wear a condom.

There was also retreat on public openness about AIDS. After I announced my own HIV status in April 1999, I was optimistic that other figures in public positions would soon speak out too about themselves. So confident was I about this – and so persistent were the rumours that cabinet members and other leading public figures were affected by HIV, and might be induced to speak out – that when the organisers of the 2000 conference asked me to deliver the keynote speech, I suggested that we first wait to see which high-profile political leaders might make similar announcements. In that case, I said, I would willingly waive the invitation and step back from delivering the keynote address.

But the president's openly expressed scepticism about the viral cause of AIDS cast a deep pall on all debate about AIDS. For a year and more after the Durban conference, not a single member of the cabinet would voice in public the view that HIV was indeed the cause of AIDS. The presidential spokesman, Parks Mankahlana, who died in mid-2000, was widely believed to have succumbed to AIDS. Shortly before his death, late in his disease progression – far too late – it was reported that he had started taking antiretroviral medication. The dissident document distributed within ANC circles in April 2002 (which I mention in Chapter Three) blamed Mankahlana's death on 'the antiretroviral drugs he was wrongly persuaded to consume'. It went on: 'He died prematurely, but the professionals who fed him the drugs that killed him remain free to feed others with the same drugs. They lived to tell us and the world that their patient had died of a virus they had never found in his body.'

114

The same document went on to ascribe the death of twelve-year-old Nkosi Johnson – a brave hero, rescued by his adoptive mother Gail Johnson from an almost certain death in infancy, whose speech at the opening of the Durban conference contained a moving testament to the suffering stigma had caused him – also to 'the antiretroviral drugs he was forced to consume': 'The pain of his unnecessary death, and the undignified media pictures of his suffering, were a platform that was used to market precisely the drugs that killed this child.'

An appalled chill fell over discussion everywhere.

The government's response became visibly hobbled with ambivalence and uncertainty. The first in-principle willingness it showed to contemplate publicly providing antiretroviral medicines in any form was in April 2002. This was five months after treatment activists led by the Treatment Action Campaign had obtained an order in the Pretoria High Court requiring that government supply antiretroviral medications to pregnant mothers to prevent HIV transmission to their children. In an historic judgment, the Constitutional Court in July 2002 confirmed the essence of the High Court's order.

The Constitutional Court's judgment built on the foundations the court had laid in an earlier case that an individual living with HIV who had suffered discrimination brought against the national airline. Just three months after the Durban conference, the court prohibited irrational discrimination against job-seekers with AIDS or HIV. The medical issues were undisputed on appeal. But, tellingly, the court went out of its way to engage in an exercise in public education. Its judgment set out in pointed detail the scientific evidence that proved that HIV is the cause of AIDS.

This part of the airline judgment proved prescient. Eighteen months later the nevirapine case confronted the court with one of its largest challenges since the transition to democracy – the government's refusal to introduce a national programme to counter the transmission of HIV from pregnant mothers to their infants. Although exhaustively documented evidence supported the efficacy, attainability and simple monetary good sense of such programmes – leaving aside the humane imperative for them – and even though the drugs were offered free to it, the government refused to implement such a programme.

The denialist shadow seemed to loom large behind the government's resistance. In its court papers and in argument before the courts, the government justified its refusal by claiming the drugs were toxic – a tenet central to the entire conspiratorialist theory of the AIDS denialists.

The Constitutional Court brushed aside this argument. Invoking its earlier exposition of the causes of AIDS, it pointed out that the evidence established that drug safety was 'no more than a hypothetical issue'. It held that there was no evidence to suggest that a dose of the antiretroviral drug in question (nevirapine) to both mother and child at the time of birth would result in any harm to either of them.

Observing that AIDS was 'the greatest threat to public health in our country', the Court ruled that South Africa's visionary democratic constitution demanded that government act decisively on the MTCT issue. It granted an order requiring government to devise and implement within its available resources 'a comprehensive and co-ordinated programme to realise progressively the rights of pregnant women and their newborn children to have access to health services to combat mother-to-child transmission of HIV'.

The Constitutional Court's order did not oblige the government to provide only nevirapine to combat perinatal transmission of HIV. The Court expressly stated in paragraph 4 of its orders that its rulings 'do not preclude government from adapting its policy in a manner consistent with the constitution if equally appropriate or better methods become available to it for the prevention of mother-to-child transmission'. Government was in the meantime, however, directed to make nevirapine or any other appropriate drug available to women wanting it.

Studies later confirmed what was already known, namely that the single-dose nevirapine regimen results in nevirapine-resistant strains being detected in a significant minority of women. This renders nevirapine less useful for inclusion in later full-scale combination therapy for these women. Indeed, using nevirapine in conjunction with other antiretrovirals more effectively reduces transmission than the single-dose regimen. Seizing on the recent publication of study results, Health Minister Manto Tshabalala-Msimang was reported to have stated at the Bangkok international AIDS conference in July 2004 that the government had been prematurely 'forced' into providing nevirapine before it had completed its research. If so, the statement was erroneous: the court order embodied no such constraint.

Since the Constitutional Court judgment, tens of thousands of mothers and children have received the single-dose nevirapine regimen in South Africa. It is beyond rational question that thousands of young lives and immeasurable suffering have been spared.

The Constitutional Court is perhaps South Africa's most successful institution of the democratic transition. Its members, now largely black, enjoy huge respect, together with its judgments. The Court is sympathetic to the government's social and democratic (as opposed to its purely party political) aims. On AIDS it used its stature wisely and restrainedly, but with unmistakable power.

Its judgments showed that irrationality and obfuscation had no place in South Africa's response to the dire AIDS threat. It directed the government onto a road that, if followed, would lead to the effective and coherent national response to the epidemic that was then so tragically lacking. Most importantly, its order implied the simple fact that human intervention can save real lives and curtail real suffering. In an epidemic in which there is much dispiritedness, this came as an inspirational challenge.

President Mbeki has never publicly stated that his view is that HIV does not cause AIDS. What he has done is to ask how a virus can cause a syndrome, and to emphasise that AIDS cannot be attributed 'solely and exclusively' to HIV. He has made it plain that he regards the syndrome of immune collapse afflicting central and southern Africa as a disease 'of poverty and underdevelopment', rather than a viral syndrome for which the first-line treatment must be antiretroviral medication.

Scientists and philosophers have long debated the different roles that behaviour, physiology, environment and contagion play as sources of disease. The recognition that social factors create and help spread disease was an enlightening and humanising breakthrough in a world in which, just a few centuries back, illness was often blamed on sin and sloth. More recently, scientific breakthroughs in medical bacteriology and virology have brought further enlightenment. Science has helped us to humanise our responses to disease and to sick people, steering us away from moral blame and censorious inaction in the face of suffering.

But AIDS rekindled the passion – and the anger – in all these debates. The censorious moralists saw (and some still see) HIV disease not as the product of an infectious pathogen, but as stemming from the infected person's own reprehensible conduct. 'Sex as sin' played a large part in the early social understanding of the disease. The result was that those with HIV infection or AIDS were blamed for their own condition – as though to have sex merits the punishment of the terrible anguish of AIDS-related diseases and death.

It is a cruel and unexpected paradox that moralism of a related – and perhaps even more destructive – kind has also cut deeply into rational debate about AIDS in Africa. The claim that the conventional view on AIDS stigmatises Africans as sex-mad fiends has its source in moralistic premises similar to those that blame persons with AIDS for having contracted their condition sexually. In parallel with early moralistic responses to AIDS, African denialism also disputes that HIV is simply the product of an infectious pathogen. Wrongly attributing to the scientific approach the view that the epidemic stems from the reprehensible conduct of those infected with HIV, it rages against an imputed moralism and the stigma deriving from it. In this it refocuses obsessively on questions of moral blame for infection – precisely what AIDS workers for twenty years sought to counter.

The object of those casting doubt on the conventional causal theory of AIDS may have been to save Africans from the supposedly stigmatising effect of a Western disease model that seemed to imply that Africans' sexual conduct led to distinctive disease patterns on this continent. Yet the effect of their dissident stance was to re-stigmatise the disease.

Paradoxically, it was those advancing denialist dogma in Africa who re-moralised AIDS and re-stigmatised the disease, through their preoccupation with the sexual transmission of HIV and by suggesting that scientific epidemiology implied a moral rebuke to Africans' sexual conduct.

Yet medical science cannot and should not be all-prevailing. The epidemic has also rekindled resistance to doctors who, spurred by scientific successes, triumphantly assert that science and its products are all that humankind needs. Attacks on the 'medicalisation' of AIDS come from many sources, with different agendas. Many of them find deserving targets. 'Full lifestyle theorists' argue that there is more to getting HIV – and to falling ill with AIDS, and to recovering from AIDS – than just a virus. They accept the need for medication, but say that medication is not enough. In this they are surely right.

Social reformers also rightly urge that science is not enough. They plead for a broad, political, social and community response to the causes and management of all diseases, including AIDS. They accept the need for medication, but point out that on its own it is not enough. They, too, are right.

These points of view have in common their rejection of a purely medical model of disease causation, progression and treatment – and of a purely medical model of the social modelling (epidemiology) of disease. Their insights are essential, and they are correct. Drugs are necessary. But they are not enough.

Had it stood alone, the AIDS dissidents' emphasis on environmental factors would have enriched the debate about what causes and hastens disease in Africa. Poverty manifestly exacerbates all African pathologies, and excessive reliance on medical interventions can be a dangerous distraction from broader, more long-lasting social solutions. And President Mbeki's emphasis on the broader context of Africa's ailments is part of a heroic campaign against a grossly unjust economic world order, which holds Africa captive to its history of colonialist exploitation. His historic legacy might yet lie in his leadership of this broader campaign, with its insistence that the world should acknowledge the burdens of racism and colonialism that African economies and African people are still forced unjustly to bear.

But the conventional approach to AIDS does not dispute that diseases have environmental triggers. Nor does it deny that poverty, malnutrition, poor healthcare and adverse living conditions hasten their onset. Still less does it suggest that antiretroviral treatment can succeed in isolation. A malnourished, untended patient, living in a shack and beset with other infections, cannot benefit from antiretroviral treatment alone. She is entitled to broader social opportunities and interventive remedies – including food and housing and clean water and medical care. The South African constitution recognises this, and the government has achieved significant progress in the ten years since democracy in improving living conditions and opportunities for poor people.

So what is the difference between the AIDS denialists and those who approach AIDS conventionally? It is elementary, and it is irreducible. It concerns not the question of whether medications are sufficient – for everyone agrees that they aren't. It concerns the question whether they are necessary at all. The conventionalists' argument has been misrepresented as suggesting that Africa's only need is that boxes of pills be freighted in. That is a silly misrepresentation. The struggle in South Africa since 1999 has not been to secure antiretroviral drugs as the sole solution to HIV disease, but to ensure that they form an appropriate part of government's overall response.

The real issue in the debate was whether the denialists, who ascribe AIDS exclusively or preponderantly to environmental factors, conceded that there was any role for pills at all.

But the lives of hundreds of thousands of affluent, well-attended gay men in North America and Western Europe and elsewhere, now dead from AIDS, bear testimony to the insufficiency of environmental explanations. These men, many of whom did not take the drugs or attend the parties or have the sexually transmitted diseases the AIDS dissidents claim explain their deaths, had all the environmental privileges the world economy still systematically withholds from poor Africans. Yet they died. Their deaths testify to the terribly destructive effects of a single virus.

On the scientific and medical approach to AIDS, if every social ill were instantly removed from Africa – poverty, malnutrition, malaria, tuberculosis, polluted drinking water, lack of healthcare, warfare, migration, dislocation – there would still be an epidemic of AIDS. There would still be perhaps thirty million lives – perhaps more, perhaps fewer – at risk of a hideous, protracted disease-ridden death. There would still be perhaps thirty million people who would need antiretroviral drugs within the next decade or so to deal with the fatal effects of a virus within their bodies. There would still be thirty million people – perhaps fewer – whom no amount of environmental alleviation or 'upliftment' would save from the effects of just one virus.

There is in other words an ineradicably microbial element to AIDS. The environment alone cannot explain it, and environmental interventions alone cannot take it away. Part of the solution must therefore be microbiological. And it is medical microbiology that has produced the drugs that have near-miraculously contained the epidemic in the west; and that can hugely alleviate its hideous effects on lives and health and development in Africa.

The conventional, scientifically warranted approach to AIDS recognises the environment and concedes that medical treatment alone is not enough. But it insists that unless medical treatment is part of the overall solution, AIDS will continue to exact an appalling toll in Africa. It is here that the AIDS dissidents part company with reason and evidence. They insist that microbiology forms no essential part of a rational approach to AIDS. They blame African AIDS on the environment alone, and contest the existence and medical manageability of HIV.

It is a deeply pessimistic view: one that has not only re-stigmatised our understanding of the disease, but that has disempowered our understanding of our own capacity, as Africans, to intervene with immediate efficacy to stop appalling suffering. Science, and reason, enable us to do better.

I speak – I must speak: my life forces me to speak – with sombre passion about this. I nearly became one of the dead. After a poverty-ridden childhood, my white skin earned me passage into a relatively affluent South African adulthood. I did not party or take drugs or have multiple exposure to the seminal deposits of innumerable sexual partners. I led the generally cautious life of a hard-working lawyer. Yet I fell ill from AIDS. I fell ill from a single virus. It was transmitted to me in a single, incautious episode of unprotected receptive sexual intercourse during Easter 1985. Poverty, the environment and decadent behaviour cannot explain my illness. The virus in my body, the reality of whose presence and activity the most sophisticated medical tests monitor, overcame my affluent living circumstances and my cautious conduct. A single virus brought me to the point of near-fatal illness from AIDS.

It is only because of medical microbiology and its antiretroviral interventions that I am living today. To live is to know. It is to feel the joy of life's forces coursing through one's veins. To survive AIDS is to feel the joy of escape, and the elation of continued life. It is also to bear the duty to speak, and the responsibility to bear witness.

5 | A judge is called as witness to AIDS

In the first heady years of South Africa's democracy, as the epidemic gathered force, leaders in AIDS policy joined the throngs jostling for President Mandela's precious attention. During the negotiations leading up to the democratic transition, he had after all lent his personal impress to the development of a nonpartisan national approach to AIDS. In October 1992, he launched an initiative that joined ANC-aligned health professionals and policy-makers with officials of the outgoing apartheid government in a venture to construct a comprehensive approach to AIDS.

His backing at that time was particularly telling since, shortly before, a bloody massacre in the Vaal township of Boipatong, near Sharpeville, which apartheid agents were suspected of instigating, had derailed negotiations with the outgoing government. While responsibility for the bloodshed was being investigated, the ANC called off constitutional discussions. Yet speaking just four months later at a showground venue near Soweto, during the breach in negotiations, Mandela gave his personal endorsement to the call for national co-ordination and special exertion on AIDS.

Yet after he took office in April 1994, the other calls on President Mandela's time were too many. The transition was not yet secure. The South African economy had to be rescued from the inordinate profligacy of the outgoing regime. Despite the new government's magnanimity, many privileged whites seemed insensitive to the largesse that had befallen them, and race relations remained precarious. And there was the mundane but critical and overriding task of providing jobs, water, housing, education and other services for the black majority after more than three centuries of racial exclusion.

The task was vast. No human could give attention to all of it. And then there was also the large international stage, on which Mandela justly was a larger-than-life figure. It was here, at the influential leaders' and economists' think-tank at Davos in Switzerland, that Mandela made his first significant statement on AIDS. That was in February 1997, nearly three years after he took office.

Long before, we had made strenuous efforts to enlist his immense personal stature for AIDS awareness and antidiscrimination campaigns. Soon after the democratic changeover in April 1994, my co-chair and I, leading the national convention of government, non-government, business and activist AIDS groupings (NACOSA) that had sprung from the 1992 initiative, sought urgent time with the new president to enjoin him to make AIDS a priority. We held a preliminary meeting with a senior official in the presidency, the Reverend Frank Chikane, a former head of the South African Council of Churches, who is now the head of President Mbeki's office. He listened sympathetically. But when he got back to us, it was to say that President Mandela had delegated our request for a meeting to his second deputy president, FW de Klerk. Though disappointed, we appreciated that Mandela had ensured that the issue stayed at executive level.

Our meeting with Deputy President De Klerk took place on a bright summer's morning towards the end of November 1994. In an imposing room in the executive offices in the Union Buildings in Pretoria he welcomed us in, taking his seat at the head of a massive polished wooden table. Apart from the two of us – the NACOSA co-chairs – one other official was present. It was not to be a 'set-piece' meeting, with journalists and visitors present, but a business meeting, where we could get down to a firm exchange of views and messages on a critical topic.

I had not met De Klerk before. But before the transition I had publicly censured his government for ineptitude on the epidemic and for inattention to the crisis it foretold. To too many it had seemed that the outgoing government viewed AIDS through apartheid's denigrating racial lens as a 'black' problem. Yet De Klerk was our access to the Mandela presidency, and we were determined to use every minute to ensure greater executive attention from the new leadership.

But ten minutes into our meeting it received a radical, and refreshing, enhancement. To our surprise, in strode senior Deputy President Thabo Mbeki – an unannounced and unexpected presence. He had gone out of his way to make time to join a meeting, off his schedule, that had been assigned to De Klerk. We rose in delight. The deputy president warmly embraced both me and my co-chair, Dr Clarence Mini, who had been in exile during apartheid. I had met Mbeki – then an influential member of the ANC's top leadership – in June 1988, when senior lawyers and progressive-leaning judges held exploratory constitutional talks with the still-banned liberation organisation at Nuneham Park near Oxford. The meeting, brokered by Oxford legal philosopher Ronald Dworkin, made good progress in setting out legal and constitutional space for genuine social transformation of South African society.

Taking time out from the formal meetings, Arthur Chaskalson, later Constitutional Court head and chief justice, led a handful of us to a special meeting with ANC President Oliver R Tambo at the nearby country home of liberal philanthropist David Astor. Tambo, a lion of the exiled liberation struggle, was the focus of the meeting, and we gathered respectfully around him. Before mounting repression drove him out of the country, he had been Mandela's partner in the famously named Johannesburg law firm of Mandela & Tambo.

Though Tambo presided, the most magnetic personality and intellect, both at Astor's home, and at Nuneham Park, was the organisation's rising star, Thabo Mbeki. By then it was well known that he was the 'brains' behind the ANC's creative forward engagement with South African lawyers, business people and academics. It was he who charmed business into seeing that cooperation with the ANC offered a more stable path than inaction or continued collusion with apartheid. And it was he who charmed the ANC into seeing that commitment to constitutional principle would prove more fruitful than rigid adherence to some of its past ideological precepts.

As an openly gay judge proudly holding office under South Africa's new constitution, I had particular reason to appreciate the determination that Thabo Mbeki had shown to include a generous conception of African humanity in South Africa's future vision of itself. In 1987, a senior ANC member in London, Mrs Ruth Mompati, had made unreflective comments about gays and lesbians, suggesting that they were all moneyed whites who did not need constitutional protection to secure equality. Anti-apartheid groupings in Holland and Scandinavia, who had supported the ANC steadily through years of exile, responded with dismay – a feeling I shared as a gay leader within South Africa who was also deeply committed to anti-apartheid legal reform. It was Thabo Mbeki who intervened decisively to save the situation. He issued a public statement on behalf of the exiled organisation recording a munificent assurance that the ANC's conception of legal equality embraced all groups who had experienced discrimination under apartheid, including gays and lesbians.

By an almost certain causal sequence, assisted by the stand that brave leaders like Simon Nkoli had taken, that assurance was translated during the transitional negotiations into ANC support for express mention of sexual orientation as a protected condition under the new constitution. And further along the same causal line I surely owed my own judicial appointment as an openly gay man to the humanising, expansive conception of Africa that Mbeki espoused.

Now, a short few years after his London intervention on the gay and lesbian debate, he sat as deputy president in the Union Buildings, listening intently as my colleague and I emphasised the severity of the problem, and the necessity for AIDS to become a governmental priority in every sphere. His responses left no doubt that for him AIDS was a central and arresting issue. We left hopeful. If we could not get to President Mandela himself, we had nevertheless had the benefit of real engagement with the most imposing intellect in government.

But within a few years, certain dogmas of AIDS dissidence seemed somehow to have gained perhaps irremovable purchase in South Africa's struggle with AIDS. Denialist attitudes appeared to be behind the hideous wavering of the South African leadership on the issue of drug treatment in the critical years of 2000, 2001 and 2002. Only in August 2003 did the government finally say that it would gear up to provide antiretroviral drugs through the public health services – a step much poorer, far less resourced African countries had taken long years before.

Right until the surprise announcement, many feared that a pub-

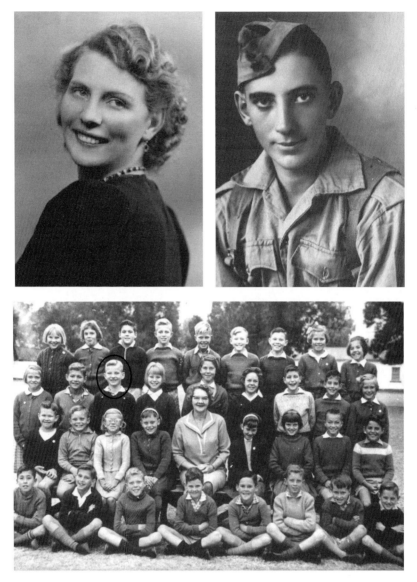

TOP LEFT: Salomé Schoeman, photographed in Bloemfontein in about 1946 or 1947, shortly before her marriage to Kenneth Hughson Cameron.

TOP RIGHT: Kenneth Hughson Cameron, father to Jeanie and me, painfully young and strikingly handsome, in uniform while fighting Nazism during World War II.

BOTTOM: The Standard One class at the Presbyterian Children's Home Primary School in Queenstown.

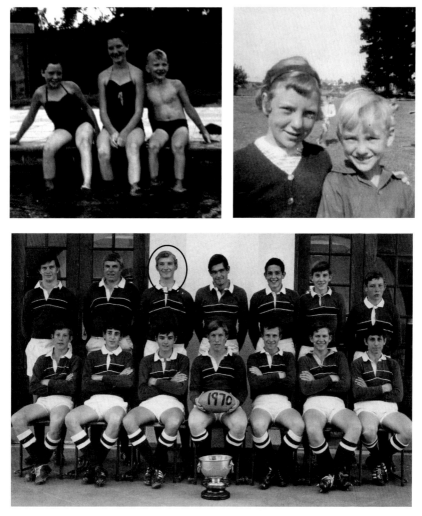

TOP LEFT: With Laura and Jeanie at a Johannesburg poolside a week before Laura's death.

TOP RIGHT: Jeanie's arm around me at the Queenstown children's home in the winter after Laura's death, 1961.

BOTTOM: Rugby team at Pretoria Boys' High School, 1970.

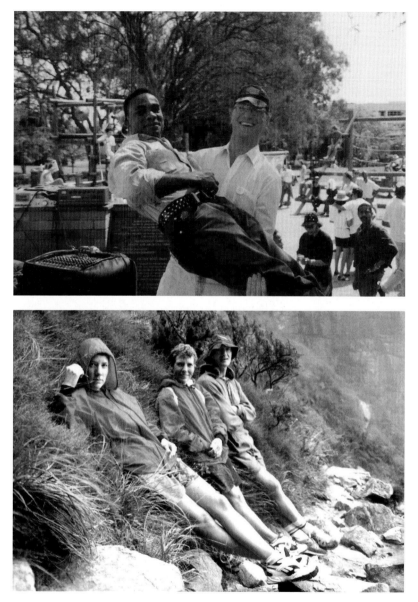

TOP: Gay and Lesbian Pride – my last before becoming a judge – Johannesburg, September 1994.

BOTTOM: Climbing Table Mountain, Cape Town, with Jeanie and Marlise on 10 December 1997, one month after starting anti-retroviral treatment. (photograph: Wim Richter)

TOP: With my mother Sally and Jeanie at Sally's 80th birthday in January 2001, ten months before Sally's death.

BOTTOM: As Wits Council Chairperson, capping my niece Marlise Richter at her graduation, April 1999.

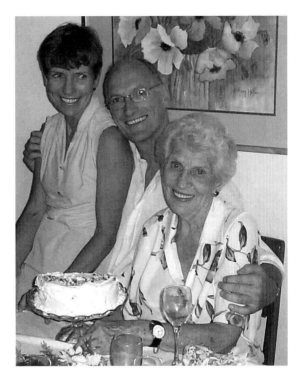

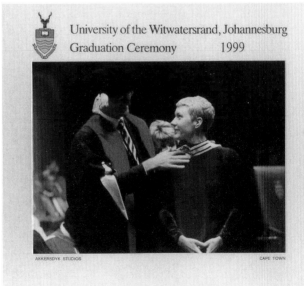

University of the Witwatersrand, Johannesburg
Graduation Ceremony   1999

AKKERSDYK STUDIOS   CAPE TOWN

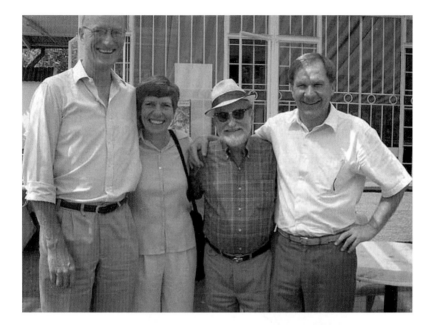

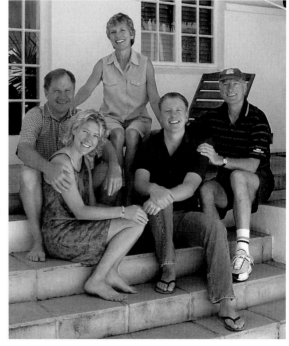

TOP: With Jeanie and her husband Wim Richter and Prof Phillip Tobias at Wits University's Sterkfontein World Heritage site, February 2002.

BOTTOM: On holiday with the Richters in Camps Bay, Cape Town, December 2004. (photograph: Andrea Scheepers)

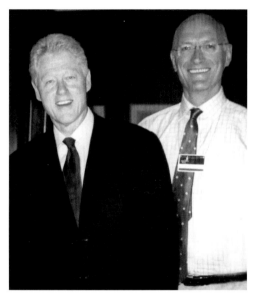

With former president Bill Clinton at Rhodes House, Oxford, during the Centenary Reunion of Rhodes Scholars, July 2003.

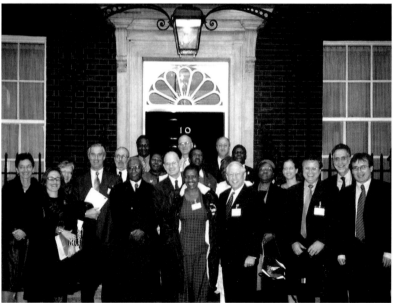

Outside No 10 Downing Street, London, with five African health ministers and other leaders on 21 November 2003 after meeting in the Cabinet Room on AIDS with Prime Minister Tony Blair, Secretary of State for Overseas Development Hillary Benn, President George W Bush, Secretary of State Colin Powell and National Security Advisor Condoleeza Rice. (photograph: Bill Roedy)

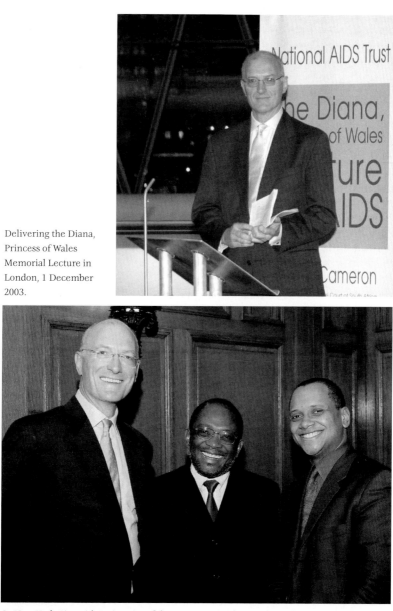

Delivering the Diana, Princess of Wales Memorial Lecture in London, 1 December 2003.

In New York City with University of the Witwatersrand Vice-Chancellor Loyiso Nongxa and Newsweek Chief of Correspondents Marcus Mabry (a friend from his Johannesburg stint as Africa Bureau Chief) on a fund-raising trip for Wits in February 2004.

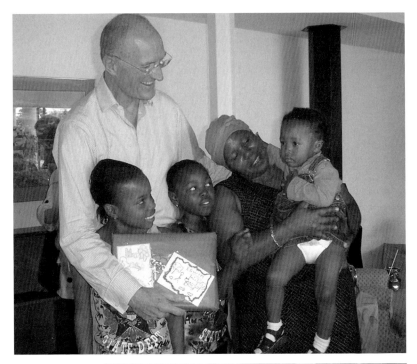

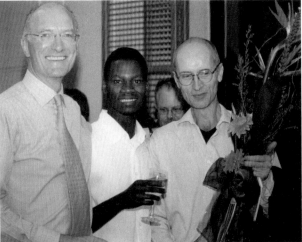

TOP: Receiving birthday gifts from Sophie Kekana, Diana, Paulina and Angela, February 2004.

BOTTOM: With friends Khopotso Bodibe and Timothy Trengove Jones after speaking at a Wits University book launch, 31 March 2004. (Photograph: Sabelo Mlangeni)

lic programme of antiretroviral provision might never form part of government's AIDS response: that the scepticism induced by AIDS denialism might have taken root so firmly in the upper echelons of government that antiretroviral treatment would remain anathema. Fortunately that was not to be. But the change was not easily wrought. It took concentrated work by many leaders and opinion-formers and AIDS activists (led by the Treatment Action Campaign). It also took the colossus-like intervention of former President Mandela.

Seven years after the meeting at the Union Buildings with deputy presidents Mbeki and De Klerk, I received a significant call. On one of the first few days of December 2001, my telephone at my office at the law school of the University of the Witwatersrand rang. Across the line came the unmistakably distinctive tones of former President Mandela. Did I have time to come and see him? It was rather urgent. He wondered if I could make myself available to discuss an important and delicate matter privately with him. He did not want to impose on what he knew was my busy schedule. (The former president speaks with such generous civility that it is at times impossible not to conclude that he enjoys gently teasing one.)

The next evening I went to his home in Houghton, Johannesburg. In his living room he took his seat in a large armchair and gestured me to sit on his right, where he could hear best. Apart from two little boys who bustled in to say goodnight to their grandfather, we were alone. Madiba wanted to talk about AIDS, and about ways in which he could help ensure a response that would save lives in our country. Though the former president spoke with tactful allusiveness, two things seemed very clear to me: he would do nothing to impair or impugn the authority and standing of his successor; but he would play an unequivocal part in asserting the vital significance of securing antiretroviral treatment as part of the remedy for the growing numbers of those dying from AIDS in South Africa.

As I was leaving, Madiba made a special request. Would I let him have a personal statement that set out the facts relating to AIDS as they had affected my life? I drafted it that evening, and took it to him the next day. He also asked me to call Professor William Makgoba, to pass on a request that he should similarly pay a call at the

Houghton house. From the car I phoned the professor immediately. He was in Cape Town: he flew to Johannesburg the next day. On his way to Madiba, he stopped off at my home.

It was evident to both of us that Madiba would make a significant intervention on AIDS. During his presidency I had criticised his leadership on the issue. Now it was plain that, at the age of 83, he was deliberately assuming responsibility for an entirely new and unforeseen task – to assert the need, within the ANC and more widely, for antiretroviral treatment to form part of the government's overall response to AIDS. It was clear that his intervention would be momentous. Perhaps it would be he who could set right the anguished debate about AIDS in our country.

I spoke to almost no one about my meeting. But eight months later, in his closing address at the Barcelona AIDS conference in July 2002, Madiba himself told delegates how he had called me in and discussed my antiretroviral regimen with me. His public statements on AIDS, starting in December 2001, added his massive moral stature to pleas for rationality in the debate about antiretroviral treatment in dealing with AIDS in South Africa. Within a few months of our meeting, Mandela awarded the Nelson Mandela Prize for Health and Human Rights to two University of the Witwatersrand researchers, Prof James McIntyre and Dr Glenda Gray, who have played a leading role in researching and introducing peri-natal HIV transmission strategies to Africa. As a past winner of the award, I had the privilege of being flown down to the smart Mount Nelson Hotel in Cape Town on Thursday 7 February to hear him speak. The next day, just a few hundred metres away, Parliament was to open and President Mbeki was to deliver his state of the nation address. The juxtaposition seemed significant.

What many suspected in Madiba's choice of date and venue became unmistakable as he delivered his address. It was classic Madiba – lighthearted, passionate, elliptical and plain-speaking, all the same time. He lauded McIntyre and Gray, and spoke with sombre intensity about the plight of mothers and babies with HIV. Then, as often in a Mandela speech, he became personal:

'Many of you will know well that some time last year I was diagnosed to be . . . [pause] Are you listening? I was diagnosed to be a cancer sufferer. I was shocked. And then there was a dispute among the various urologists in the country. My urologist who operated on me in prison said, "You must have your hormone and radio therapy". Others said, "No, this man is too old to have radio therapy", and this debate raged. I said to both groups, "You must come together and resolve this debate." They did come together at the University of Wits but they could not agree. Then I said, "Now you come and have this debate in front of me", and they came. Of course I couldn't follow the technical terms at all and I said, "Now I've listened to you, thank you." Now they spelt out in detail the problems I'm going to have if I have a combination of the hormone as well as the radio therapy, but I am confident in my urologist and those who supported him. And when the dissidents were gone, I wondered whether it was proper for me to undergo this treatment.'

He went on to describe how he had taken the treatment despite the risk that 'doctors can make a mistake'. And yet now, as a result of treatment, he was clear of cancer: the medical intervention, supported by non-dissident medical science, had triumphed. Madiba's parable was personal and powerful: when life is at stake, trust medical science, even when debate may rage; ignore dissidents; choose reason and hope above scepticism. It was powerful and suggestive advice.

A few months later, shortly after leaving Barcelona in July 2002, Madiba paid a pointed visit to Treatment Action Campaign leader Zackie Achmat at his home in Muizenberg. Though increasingly vulnerable himself to HIV-related illnesses, Zackie had pledged not to take the drugs until they were available to everyone. Madiba went to cheer him. He also went to exhort Zackie to take the drugs. This Zackie eventually started doing just more than a year later, shortly after the government's August 2003 pledge that it would provide antiretroviral treatments through the public health services.

Before his visit to Zackie concluded, Madiba donned the now internationally famous T-shirt Zackie had designed. Emblazoned 'HIV POSITIVE', it has become far beyond South Africa's borders a symbol of the struggle for justice and reason and openness in the AIDS debate. It is worn casually and widely by many thousands of people – positive and negative – in marches, on the street, at work and at home. It has done more to lessen stigma than innumerable speeches and workshops and think-tanks. It says, as the Danish king did in the fable of the yellow star during the Nazi persecution of the Danish Jews: we all bear this condition. We are all HIV POSITIVE. We all need treatment to be made available.

Madiba too. His smiling famous features atop the white cotton HIV POSITIVE T-shirt may have marked a turning point in our national struggle about the meaning of AIDS. Perhaps it was his intervening moral voice that made the change in the government's resistance to antiretroviral drugs inevitable.

For the debate about antiretroviral drugs and the causes of AIDS was not a minor political skirmish or a difference in policy or emphasis. It was a debate literally about life and death. It was a debate about how our new democracy dealt with truth. And it involved fundamental and troubling questions about truth-telling in our new society. How we handled it would surely determine how we as a nation grappled with other, equally profound, issues of truth.

Soon after the 2002 Barcelona AIDS conference, the General Council of the Bar of England and Wales (the barristers' professional society in London) invited me to a special award ceremony at the Bar's annual conference in London. In the atmosphere of increasing crisis at home, as AIDS deaths mounted and the government still appeared to be prevaricating about the very existence of the epidemic, and about whether it would ever contemplate providing antiretroviral treatment as part of its programme, I chose as my theme for the award dinner the role that law and legal reasoning can play in countering untruth.

Law is often weak, I said. But where its processes are strong, it can play an inestimable role in exposing illogicality and untruth. I spoke about a recent London High Court judgment against a famous historian who had propagated lies about the Nazi murder of Jews during the Second World War. The judgment of Sir Charles Gray, the High Court judge who dismissed David Irving's defamation claim against a Jewish historian who called him anti-Semitic, exposed Irving as a 'Holocaust denier' – one who unscrupulously denied the truth about the systematic murder of millions of Jews in Nazi Germany.

And I drew a partial parallel with the two judgments the South African Constitutional Court had delivered on AIDS – the one deftly but unmistakably affirming the rational cause-and-effect connection between HIV and AIDS; the other quietly insisting that antiretroviral treatment was a basic right for pregnant mothers who wanted to save their babies from HIV, and a necessary part of the nation's response to the epidemic.

I went on to make a point about systems of knowledge and belief and disbelief. I compared those who systematically deny the Nazi Holocaust of World War II as an historical fact, and those who systematically deny the epidemic of HIV-caused disease as an historical and current fact. The one type of knowledge refutation I called 'Holocaust denialism', the other 'AIDS denialism'. I observed that the two belief systems were strikingly similar in the way they operated to deny established fact.

To deny something is to refuse to admit its truth or existence. In psychology, ordinary 'denial' has a well-known meaning. It is a defence mechanism involving a refusal to acknowledge an intolerable truth or emotion. This sort of 'denial' is common. It underlies many personal and political responses to the AIDS epidemic. At a personal level, many people believe themselves immune to infection. Once infected, they convince themselves that they are exempt from passing on the virus. Or they convince themselves that they will never fall ill.

This common form of 'denial' I have experienced in my own life. Though cognitively accepting that I was infected with HIV, I continued – even as the evidence mounted that I was falling sick – to hope against hope that I would never fall ill with AIDS. Despite the unmistakable signals from blood tests that warned that my immune defences were failing, and that my viral load was rising, I hoped against belief and probability that somehow I would escape. That (together with fear of treatment failure, plus the prohibitive expense) was why I postponed starting on medication until I fell severely ill in late 1997 and had no choice.

This sort of ordinary 'denial' occurs also at a political level. In newly democratic South Africa, the onset of a mass epidemic of virally borne and sexually transmitted disease and death, amidst all the other traumas besetting Africa, seemed unjust, intolerable, unimaginable. So 'denial' in this common psychological sense was to be expected in South Africa. Indeed, it manifested itself also in many African countries, where in the early years AIDS figures were suppressed and the impact of the epidemic denied. Uganda later led the way out of political denial of the AIDS epidemic into openness and acceptance.

But ordinary psychological 'denial', which we all experience and suffer from, is very different from denial as a systematic form of knowledge refutation. That is 'denial' in its dogmatic form. It is the latter variety of systematic denial that the AIDS dissidents espouse. Psychological denial may underlie or help to explain AIDS dissidence. Yet the two are very different. Those who are in ordinary 'denial' about AIDS – whether personally or politically – are unable emotionally to admit or act upon the fact of HIV infection or AIDS illness. They do not try logically or factually to refute the epidemic. Their desire is to avoid, not disprove, the facts. They want to postpone acceptance and action rather than to controvert the need for action altogether.

Dogmatic AIDS denialism is quite different. It is not a subjective defence against pain (though of course pain may in part explain the need for it). It is an attack against objective truth. It involves the systematic refusal, for preconceived reasons of doctrine, to accept the evidence that HIV exists as a virally borne, sexually transmitted fact. It sets out systematically to refute the existence of AIDS as an epidemic manifestation of a medically treatable condition.

Inflexible presuppositions underlie dogmatic AIDS denialism. These impel dissidents to reject the facts regardless of the evidence establishing them. Denialists find the facts simply unacceptable. So they set out to render them untrue. Their tools are quasi-rationalist methods of argument, evasion and distortion.

I suggested in my talk to the English barristers that in substance, method and motive, AIDS denialism showed striking parallels to Holocaust denialism. Both are systems of knowledge refutation. In substance, both deny facts that others generally accept as proven on the basis of massive and overwhelming evidence. In the one case, the dissidents deny an historical fact – the calculated destruction of European Jewry. In the other, they deny a current fact – a virally borne, sexually transmitted epidemic that is devastating central and southern Africa.

In method, both use dubious and evasive methods to distort, conceal and evade the truth. Both exploit the undisputed fact that certain data are either indeterminate (unascertained) or indeterminable (not capable of being ascertained). Thus, no one knows precisely how many Jews died in the Holocaust. Responsible estimates by reputable Holocaust historians vary hugely. Some Jewish historians have estimated that the number of Jews who died in the Nazi Holocaust may be as low as three million. The usual estimate is much higher: between five and six million.

No one will ever know. The precise number of Jews and gypsies and homosexuals who together with others died in the Nazi death camps can never be determined. Holocaust denialists use this indeterminability to cast doubt on whether any systematic murder of Jews took place at all. They exploit the indeterminacy of the figures to suggest that Jewish historians exaggerate them for political gain.

AIDS dissidents in Africa have resorted to a strikingly similar strategy. They point out that the reach and scope of the epidemic in Africa is uncertain. That fact is undeniable. In fact, the size of the African epidemic can never be made certain. The precise numbers of Africans dead or dying from AIDS, the numbers of those with HIV who risk death from AIDS, are indeterminable. Dissidents use this uncertainty to stoke doubt about whether the epidemic exists at all, or to cast doubts on its extent or its significance.

The comparison becomes particularly illuminating, I argued, when one considers how denialists in each camp impute motives to their opponents. Holocaust denialists have to offer some explanation for the fact that many thousands of apparently respectable, scrupulous and honest scholars – historians and scientists – assert, and persist in asserting, that millions of Jews died in the Nazi concentration camps. The same applies to the thousands of scientists and epidemiologists and health workers who claim that a calamitous epidemic of death and suffering is taking place in central and southern Africa because of a viral, sexually transmitted infection.

Why would such numbers of seemingly respectable persons tell such lies? Dogmatists in both camps say that most of these people are dupes – herd-followers with no independent means of thinking. Happy to repeat conventional 'truths' without examining the evidence afresh, they cling to mass thinking because it is easier and more convenient – and because it secures their jobs and income. But this is surely not enough. Truth and falsehood are established by contestation – by vigorous debate in which the evidence for and against a proposition is examined, re-examined and eventually judged provisionally sufficient or provisionally wanting. This is how 'paradigms' shift. In the case of both the Nazi Holocaust and AIDS in Africa, the premises of the factual assertions have been thoroughly contested. And the evidence for each – one a horror of history, one a continuing calamity – stands. By all rational methods of inference and knowledge acquisition, there was a Nazi Holocaust against the Jews, and there is a sexually transmitted epidemic devastating central and southern Africa.

Yet the dissidents in each camp dispute this. They have quasi-rationalist refutations of all the evidence that historians, camp survivors, virologists, epidemiologists and doctors can bring. Their own belief system requires an explanation of why their opponents so fiercely persist in clinging to what they say is falsehood.

In both cases, the dissidents say, there is a conspiracy underlying it all. The 'facts' are manufactured and propagated by a group of people with a hidden intent. What is that intent? In both cases, the dissidents see the answer in racist thinking. They invoke a form of racial conspiracy. Holocaust deniers ascribe the assertion of the 'falsehood' that millions of Jews were systematically murdered under Hitler to a clique of Jewish historians and politicians, aided and abetted by thousands of others, whose ultimate design is to exercise influence over – or better still control – the world.

In its African form, AIDS denialists say that the conventional medical and scientific approach to AIDS (that it is a virally caused, sexually transmitted disease that should be medically treated with antiretroviral drugs) stems ultimately from a Western corporate conspiracy to peddle drugs to poor Africans. They claim (although there is no evidence for this) that the markets for antiretrovirals in the West are declining. So new markets must be created in Africa: Africans suffering from the environmental effects of poverty and malnutrition and poor healthcare must be made to take unnecessary drugs so that corporations can continue to garner extortionate profits, and so that bureaucrats in Geneva and elsewhere can keep their cushy jobs.

The jobs of thousands of scientists, doctors, researchers and medical technologists depend on the existence of the AIDS epidemic in Africa. They must continue to claim that it exists, even though the evidence for it (the dissidents say) is flawed and false. Underlying it all is a racist conspiracy to demean Africans by impugning their sexual dignity, and to exploit them by selling useless and toxic medications to them. Ultimately, the white racist conspirators' design – the African AIDS denialists say – is to poison and kill Africans.

This was the view that seemed to have high authority in South Africa during the nightmare years of AIDS denialism. As many thousands of South Africans were falling sick and dying, it was the view that seemed to underlie government's scepticism about and resistance to providing antiretroviral medication to the public.

If this was so, I thought, the peril was such that the matter required clear and trenchant public debate.

Six months after my London speech, I expanded and developed this theme more formally in a special lecture I was invited to give at Harvard Law School's Human Rights Program in April 2003. Just after I returned from an icy Massachusetts – where an unseasonably late snowfall had caught me improvidently coatless – the lecture attracted the attention of Mondli Makhanya, who then edited South Africa's influential high-brow weekly, the *Mail & Guardian* (he is now the youngest-ever editor of the mass-circulation Johannesburg *Sunday Times*).

Mondli decided to run the lecture as the main front-page spread for the *M&G's* Easter edition. He and two senior editorialists, Nawaal Deane and Ferial Haffajee (who succeeded Mondli as editor when he went to the *Sunday Times*) excerpted it very fully and carefully, running most of its text over nearly three pages. The heading he chose was 'The Dead Hand of Denialism'.

The copy made sombre Easter reading. It spoke about President Mbeki's silence on the causes and treatment of AIDS. 'He rarely speaks

135

about AIDS at all – itself a cause for comment in a country where the official governmental statistics service estimates that many hundreds of thousands of people are dying of AIDS each year.' It pointed out that a few months before, in January 2003, Health Minister Manto Tshabalala-Msimang had invited a prominent and vocal AIDS denialist, Dr Robert Giraldo, to address the meeting of the Southern Africa Development Community's ministerial Health Committee, which she chaired.

According to reports from the meeting, Giraldo informed the ministers that 'the transmission of AIDS from person to person is a myth'. In his view, '[t]he homosexual transmission of the epidemic in Western countries, as well as the heterosexual transmission in Africa, is an assumption made without any scientific validation'. Reports claimed that the government had retained Giraldo's services to advise it on 'nutrition'. In addition, reports had suggested that in Parliament Finance Minister Trevor Manuel had questioned the usefulness of spending public money on antiretroviral medications as 'a waste of very limited resources'.

Until September 2002, the most that the government would say was that its policies were based on the 'assumption' that HIV causes AIDS. As late as March 2003, it would not say more than that its policies were based on the 'premise' that HIV causes AIDS. My lecture strafed the life-imperilling ambiguity of these expressions. The ambivalence they revealed about the leadership's underlying commitment was, I said, all too tragically apparent. How can a deathly crisis be managed on the basis of tenuous 'hypotheses'? 'It is as if a formerly avowed racist were to undertake to treat black people on the "assumption" or "premise" that they are his equals. The insult,' I said, 'is patent.'

The epidemic of sickness, suffering and death was, I stated, gathering intensity in South Africa. About one in five adult South Africans had AIDS or HIV. Tens, indeed hundreds of thousands of South Africans were dying of AIDS. Without immediate action, millions more would follow. Despite these sombre facts, there was by April 2003 little evidence that government had taken the path of constructive and decisive action.

Apart from some brave and imaginative initiatives in the private and non-governmental sectors, and despite two important and hopeful cabinet statements in April and October 2002, a decisive national response had been 'all but paralysed'. 'There is,' I said, 'increasingly a dualism between governmental statement and action concerning AIDS.' While cabinet statements acknowledged the 'hypothesis' or 'assumption' that HIV caused AIDS, 'the evidence points to the dismal conclusion that the dead hand of denialism still weighs down all too heavily on the development of a rational and effective response to AIDS'.

'Although HIV is now a medically manageable condition, government still refuses to commit itself to a national treatment plan for AIDS – even though late last year substantial progress was made in negotiations between business, non-governmental organisations and the heads of two government departments in devising such a plan.

'With all deliberate understatement, the cost in human lives and suffering of denialist-inspired equivocation in national AIDS policy can be described only as horrendous. A leading AIDS activist, Zackie Achmat, has referred to government's policies – with resonant imagery – as "a holocaust against the poor".

'AIDS offers special challenges, not merely to the governments of Africa, but to the peoples and governments of the whole world. This is not merely because of the scale of the impending disaster, in which UNAIDS estimates that tens of millions people may die over the next half-century. It is because the disease accentuates all the other inequities in a world where some enjoy a life of unimaginable wealth, while others die unnecessary and avoidable deaths amidst remediable poverty.

'Death from AIDS is now avoidable. With carefully administered treatments, and subject to monitoring and with appropriate medical care, AIDS is no longer a fatal disease. It is now a medically manageable condition. I know this from my own life, which without those treatments would have ended three or more years ago. Neither as a person living with AIDS nor as a judge – one who holds office proudly under one of the world's most visionary constitutions – can I stand apart from the struggle for truth and for action about AIDS, and the role that lawyers and the legal system are called to play in it.'

I concluded my Harvard lecture:

'We live in a world of tumult, in which truth is contested for many reasons – to justify war, to license injustice and to conceal iniquity. Amidst the dangers of war and the hatreds of centuries, we rightly view with diffidence the contribution that the law and legal process can make in these great clashes of truth. But the modest craft of rationality that lawyers espouse, with their modest panoply of instruments, honed in the mechanisms of adversarial scrutiny, seem sharp enough to pry open untruth and distortion, and strong enough to counter irrationality of the most egregious and threatening kinds.

'The law, though of limited utility in all too many situations of injustice and untruth, becomes when well utilised amidst minimal conditions for its success an extremely powerful force.

'Both Holocaust and AIDS denial remind us of our own terrible weaknesses and vulnerabilities as humans, and of the reluctance we all feel to own them. But the struggle for truth they involve also inspires us to greater thought and action. For truth, classically, is freedom, and from freedom in truth comes the capacity to build and plan and act better. AIDS in Africa calls us to unleash that capacity.'

The publication of the bulk of the Harvard lecture in the *Mail & Guardian* instantly provoked contention. And it earned me my second attack, in less than ten years, from a minister of justice. The first attack was in 1987, when the last justice minister in the apartheid government took exception to my criticism of judges under apartheid who lent succour and support to an iniquitous system (Chapter One). Now the minister of justice in South Africa's democratic government had attacked me for speaking out, as a judge living with AIDS, about what I saw as iniquitous untruth in the debate about the disease and the proper remedies for it.

It soon became clear that the comparison I had made between the belief system created by AIDS deniers and that erected by deniers of the Nazi Holocaust had hit a raw nerve. Soon after the *M&G* appeared, a well-connected talk-show host on the national broadcast network, Eric Miyeni, invited me onto his show to discuss my lecture. I thanked him for the invitation, but felt I had to decline. I wrote to the show's producer carefully explaining this stand.

I had always tried to be careful about what speaking engagements

I accepted. My Harvard lecture was certainly contentious. It trod deep into current political controversy. But it had been delivered on a formal occasion, in an appropriate academic context, with full academic and intellectual authority to back its every assertion. It had not been delivered at a public meeting or at the hustings. Carefully footnoted and deliberately expressed, when published it would be open to proper scrutiny and refutation.

The *M&G* excerpt had been very full and careful. It had conveyed the proper gist of the lecture in its proper reasoned context. Their report, to whose publication I agreed, was anything but sensationalist. For me to go onto a radio talk show to repeat and debate and propagate the lecture's main themes would, by contrast, I thought, be wrong. It would be treading across the judicial/political divide. I would be entering a form and medium of public debate that would be inappropriate for me as a judge to engage in.

I realised, I said in my letter to the talk-show host, that it is a hard line to draw. But I had been trying truthfully to draw it.

The show would go ahead without me.

On the road after an early afternoon meeting, I listened to the Eric Miyeni show in my car. The host introduced the topic by reading from what appeared to be a lengthy prepared statement. I listened with increasing concern. Then dismay. Far from representing my argument on truth-telling about the Nazi Holocaust and the AIDS epidemic fairly, he seemed to go out of his way to distort it. Far from explaining how I had compared the methods and motivations of those who systematically deny the mass murder of Jews in Nazi Germany with those who systematically deny a virally borne epidemic of AIDS, he seemed to suppress the main point of my lecture in favour of a wildly mistaken – and grossly unfair – misrepresentation of it.

I had, the talk-show host told his listeners, compared the government's AIDS policies to the Nazi Holocaust. I had drawn a 'not so subtle comparison,' he claimed, between President Thabo Mbeki and Hitler. He told listeners that 'in effect' I had accused the president of deliberately killing people.

I listened in amazement. Not even Zackie Achmat, an outspoken and unsparing activist – who used the challenging imagery of a 'holocaust against the poor' to describe the effects of denying people treatment – has ever accused the government of deliberately killing people with AIDS. (A holocaust, as opposed to 'the Holocaust', means any mass destruction or mass death. Use of the word does not suggest that the deaths are deliberately inflicted.) Nor had Zackie ever compared the government's AIDS policies to Nazism.

What gave the talk-show host reason to believe that I had done so?

The talk-show host went on to cite detailed statistics defending the government's response to AIDS. It was, he said, one of the best AIDS policies in Africa. The government was spending millions on AIDS, and to suggest otherwise was irresponsible.

He then invited listeners to phone in with their views of my attack on the president and on the government. Without exception – of course – they called in to express their indignation. How could I compare the president to Hitler?

It seemed a carefully synchronised response to the impact the article had caused – not joining issue with its main themes, but setting out to vilify me in the public mind for an argument I had never made. Though I have given and taken in severe public debate on more than one occasion, I had to admit that I was stunned.

Back in my office, I decided I had to write to the producer and the presenter. The on-air comments were not true or accurate or fair, I wrote. They were based on a misreading of my article. 'I never made a comparison between the killing of Jews in Nazi Germany and AIDS in South Africa. Nor did I make any comparison, direct or indirect, subtle or unsubtle, intentional or unintentional, between President Mbeki and Hitler. My comparison was not between doers, but between deniers. I was not comparing perpetrators, but people who refuse to accept facts.

'The comparison I made was between the systematic refusal to accept two facts – first, the fact that Jews were deliberately killed on a huge scale in Nazi Germany (which Holocaust dissidents deny); second, the fact that AIDS is a virally transmitted infectious condition which can now successfully be treated and medically managed with antiretroviral medication (which AIDS dissidents deny). Both facts have moral significance in the modern world, which is why their denial is of great importance – and the deniers in each case use similar methods, which is why the comparison is significant.

'Mr Miyeni is of course free to differ from me on whether government's AIDS policies are in fact influenced by AIDS denialism, and he expressed himself firmly and eloquently on that. But I do not believe that, in fairness, he can say that I compared President Mbeki to Hitler. There are huge and obvious differences, the most important being that in South Africa we do not have deliberately homicidal policies but a debate about fact and truth – whether AIDS is a viral condition, mostly sexually transmitted, that can now be medically managed.

'Mr Miyeni appeared to accept that AIDS is a viral condition, caused by HIV. AIDS deniers do not. This is what my lecture was about.'

Miyeni's producer later assured me that my letter had been read out in full on the next afternoon show. I thought that the clarification would set the matter to rest. At least there had been an on-record clarification, emanating from the source of a gross misrepresentation. That, I thought, would help to set out correctly the premises of a complex and fraught debate.

This was a vain belief. But in the meanwhile I had the full-time demands of my busy 'day job' to attend to. It was the end of April. The Supreme Court of Appeal term started on 1 May. I took the four-hour car journey back to Bloemfontein, where the court sits, and gave little further thought to the talk-show rumpus. Our case list for the upcoming term was heavy. It included municipal workers' rights, copyright and trade mark infringement, employers' pension fund duties and the tricky and practically important question whether the cabinet, for purposes of discouraging fraud, had the power to bar statutory road accident compensation in cases where the vehicles involved in the accident had not actually collided with each other.

One of the cases in which I was assigned to write the lead judgment concerned a relatively rare phenomenon in our criminal courts – a double murder committed by two female co-defendants. One of the few sound criminological inferences that legal practice enables you to make is that men are the perpetrators of almost all violent crimes. But not all. These women had been sentenced to long terms of imprisonment for two gruesome and pointless murders, sparked by the erroneous belief one held that one of the victims, her deceased son's fiancée, had been responsible for his death.

The trial judge had taken fully into account the mother's distress and her depressed state after her son's puzzling suicide. What had earned her and her accomplice long prison terms (respectively 25 and 30 years in jail) was the fact that a second victim – the fiancée's sister-in-law – had been inexplicably added to the carnage. My colleagues and I concluded that the trial judge had sentenced them fairly and that the appeals could not succeed.

Another of the cases assigned to me raised a novel constitutional problem concerning the High Court's oversight relationship over the lower courts. Most of South Africa's criminal cases are dealt with by magistrates, who work under inordinate pressure in considerably less comfort than High Court judges. The fact that High Courts exercise a supervisory jurisdiction over the magistrates' courts sometimes creates practical problems, and arouses sensitivities. How to exercise the jurisdiction, particularly when magistrates appear obdurate or recalcitrant, can raise difficult issues.

In the appeal before us, a doctor in a small Eastern Cape town was arrested on a charge of raping his seventeen-year-old stepdaughter. After spending two nights in jail, he applied for bail. On accepted principles, he seemed entitled to it – as the prosecution later conceded. He was clearly not a flight risk. And he offered to leave the family home pending trial. But after hearing all the evidence the town's magistrate somewhat inexplicably postponed judgment. He told the doctor and the prosecutor that he would give his bail determination nine days later. In the meantime, the doctor would have to stay in prison. In effect, the doctor was being denied bail though the magistrate did not say so.

The doctor's lawyers urgently approached the High Court. A judge issued an order requiring the magistrate to hear argument on the bail application by three o'clock, and give judgment by four o'clock that afternoon. The magistrate did not comply. So the High Court itself granted the doctor bail. It then issued an order citing the magistrate for contempt of court in not complying with its previous order, and saddling him with a personal liability for costs.

There appeared to be some local 'sting' in the case. What it was we in the Bloemfontein appeal court did not know and could not speculate. The matter had to be decided on constitutional principle alone. (Since both doctor and magistrate were black there were no racial overtones.) The state's lawyers, arguing for the magistrate, contended that the order was intrinsically incompetent, since it interfered with the magistrate's running of his court and therefore with his judicial independence. This argument we rejected. There was well-established authority that the High Court can supervise the closest details of the magistrates' courts' functioning. On occasion, where it is necessary, the High Court must do so.

While our decision re-asserted this principle, we had to conclude that in the particular circumstances the drastic order was not warranted. What if argument was not concluded by three o'clock? Would the magistrate be in contempt of the High Court order? Rather than issuing such a detailed (and demeaning) order, we said, the High Court should simply have set aside the magistrate's order postponing judgment. This would have returned the bail application to his current roll for immediate disposal. If the magistrate then still refused to finalise the matter, the High Court had the power (which it in fact exercised) to grant bail itself.

Our decision was a compromise. But we thought it set clear lines for both magistrates and High Court judges.

Both cases – the double murder and the doctor/magistrate confrontation – involved conduct that in retrospect seemed mysterious, if not inexplicable. But the law often involves just such cases. Pondering their effect through that May term left me little time for thinking back to the talk-show host's inexplicable misrepresentation of my argument.

At the end of the court sitting in early June, I travelled to Ladybrand, a small Free State town a few hours' drive from Bloemfontein, in the picturesque mountain region bordering on Lesotho. A hospice was being opened, and the local founders had asked me to become its patron. I hoped that a mixture of occasional legal guidance and funding contacts might eventually earn me the honour of being associated with their imaginative venture. The visit gave me the opportunity to meet businessmen and lawyers for discussions on AIDS, as well as to discuss formulation of AIDS policy in Lesotho with a delegation of lawyers who specially came across for our meeting from the capital Maseru, just over the Caledon River.

Local community organisers, lawyers, business people and church leaders seemed united in the grave distress they expressed during our meetings at the toll the AIDS epidemic was taking on their communities. Any notion of debating viral causation or mortality statistics would have seemed incomprehensible, even demeaning, to the sick and to the survivors of the dead they mentioned.

The founders had ploughed exceptional vision and integrity as well as fund-raising imagination into the project. The poverty of the rural region desperately needed them all. The venture's driving force, Candy Dixie – a school contemporary from one of the raft of schools I had attended in the years after leaving the children's home – gave me some disquieting facts about how AIDS was affecting the Ladybrand community. She had started the initiative in mid-2001 when it became incontestable that AIDS was taking a toll on young adult lives and their families.

By December 2001, she said, they were caring for 43 orphans. Six months later, this had increased to 58. By December 2002, there were 96 orphans needing care. By mid-2003, when we opened the facility, the number had more than doubled, to 219. These were all bereaved children whose parents – young adults in the prime of their productive lives – had inexplicably died. Few of them, of course, had actually been diagnosed with HIV. Few of their deaths were verifiably and ascertainably due to AIDS. HIV testing was rare. But what else could explain the disquieting upward swerve in Ladybrand's young adult mortality rate? What else could account for the young children, motherless and fatherless, now needing nurture and sustenance in the public-spirited venture that was being opened?

The morning we opened the hospice, the facility's orphans marched in line and sang sweetly for us. It was a sad, sobering visit, but it was one that also inspired once again my belief in our capacity to change the epidemic and its effects by our own interventions. Ladybrand's hospice shows us that inaction and hopelessness are the least forgivable choices.

As I write this passage, on an icy Johannesburg winter's evening in mid-2004, I call Candy. She tells me that in the year since the hospice has opened, the number of AIDS orphans Hospice Ladybrand is caring for has grown by a further 50 per cent. They now number 321. By the time you read this, the number may have grown further.

Driving back to Johannesburg I pondered the chilling figures that Candy had given me. Without treatment intervention, the grim figures of dead young adults in Ladybrand would continue to increase. The lines of freshly heaped graves would expand. And the numbers of parentless orphans would continue to grow. Without immediate mass treatment provision – together, of course, with poverty alleviation, improved healthcare and attendant social improvements – Ladybrand's tragedy was being replicated in every town across South Africa.

These thoughts were interrupted by a surprising and unwelcome call. A senior legal journalist from a national newspaper had tracked me down. Did I wish to comment on the attack on me by the minister of justice in Parliament that morning?

What? An attack by the minister? What had he said?

'He has condemned you,' the journalist said, 'for comparing the government's AIDS policy to the Jewish genocide under the Nazis, and for saying that the government is like Hitler.'

But I hadn't done so!

'Well, that's what the minister has accused you of,' the journalist said: 'Would you like to comment?'

My heart sank. No, I said. I definitely had no comment to make. Giving a response could only inflame an already fraught situation. Rather, I would take it up privately, and immediately, with the minister himself. I had met him in Harare in early 1989, at a follow-up meeting to the Nuneham Park gathering six months before, where a second group of South African lawyers exploring contact with the still-banned ANC met senior figures in exile to discuss a constitutional transition. He was a warm man, impetuous at times, but not I thought unreasonable. And surely he must have taken the elementary step of reading the *M&G* article, or the lecture on which it was based, before attacking me in public? But if he had read what I had written, how could he possibly accuse me of the things he did? How could he be making the same extravagant misrepresentation that the talk-show host had made?

Returning to Johannesburg, I wrote to the minister. I referred to the press reports that reported his attack on me. If the reports were correct, I said (and I conceded that they might not be), 'I regret that the comments attributed to you are not accurately based on anything that I have ever said.'

'In April I gave a lecture at Harvard University, in which I compared systematic denial of AIDS as a virologically caused (and treatable) disease with systematic denial of the Nazi Holocaust. I never compared the government's AIDS policies to the Nazi Holocaust or the government or any of its members to Hitler.

'My lecture was excerpted in the *Mail & Guardian* of 17 April 2003. The mistaken impression that I supposedly equated the government's AIDS policies with 'Nazism', or compared the government with Hitler, may have its origin in a misrepresentation and distortion of my lecture that was broadcast on the Eric Miyeni talk show on SAfm on Thursday afternoon 24 April.

'Mr Miyeni broadcast a retraction and correction the next day. I attach the text of his correction.

'I realize that the comparison that I did draw, between different forms of systematic, ideologically based denialism, may be controversial to some people, and that my criticism of government's AIDS policies may raise genuine and important issues relating to judicial participation in politically current debates.

'I do not mind being criticised for what I have said and am more than happy to be held to account – and to defend or reconsider – what I have said. But fundamental fairness obviously requires that I should not be criticized on the basis of a distortion.

'I am very happy to be able to set any misunderstandings and misperceptions right, and therefore attach a full copy of my lecture.'

I faxed the letter and the talk-show correction, together with my Harvard lecture, to the minister's home in Sandton, Johannesburg. To be absolutely sure that he received my letter, I faxed these documents also to both his two offices, in Pretoria and Cape Town. I waited to hear from him. Yet no response came. Seventeen days later, the minister's private secretary wrote courteously to me: 'In the absence of Dr Penuell Maduna, Minister for Justice and Constitutional Development, I acknowledge receipt of your letter dated 7 June 2003. The minister is currently out of town but your letter will be brought to his attention as soon as possible after his return.'

I never heard from the minister. He had many other issues on his mind, including an investigation into alleged arms-deal corruption by his political ally, the National Director of Public Prosecutions (NDPP), Bulelani Ngcuka. Two short months later this would embroil him in controversy that would lead to the appointment of the Hefer Commission, presided over by my retired Supreme Court of Appeal colleague, Mr Justice Hefer. He later issued a report refuting allegations that during the struggle for democracy Mr Ngcuka had been a spy for the apartheid government.

The minister left office at the time of the 2004 election. He joined a leading Johannesburg law firm in a part-time capacity as a consultant. Perhaps I will see him in due course, at the sort of lawyerly gatherings that lawyers must hold and must attend. We will then I hope be able to discuss with dispassion the comparison I drew between forms of knowledge refutation. And we will be able to discuss, I hope, his understanding of the argument I made, and the issues of life and death that are at stake beneath the argument.

Did the talk-show host and the minister really understand the *Mail & Guardian* report as suggesting a comparison between Hitler's genocide and the government's AIDS policies? Many of my colleagues and friends thought not. They thought that the true comparison I had made – between historically different but methodologically similar forms of truth denial – might have been too close for comfort. Perhaps, they suggested, what I did point out about our national struggle for truth in the AIDS debate was seen to necessitate a calculated rhetorical switch to safer (if distorted) ground.

So was I set up because the challenge in the argument that I did make cut too close to the bone? I will never know. For their own understanding and representation of my argument the minister and the talk-show host will no doubt take responsibility. What matters more are the things for which I must take responsibility myself. These are primarily two. The first is for what I did say. The second is for the public position I held when I said it.

The comparison between Holocaust denial and AIDS denial was unquestionably loaded. It was more than that. It was provocative and challenging. It was not merely an intellectually ambitious comparison – albeit (I thought) carefully reasoned and justified. It was also politically contentious. It was surely inevitable that the comparison would elicit indignation and heated response.

When I made the comparison I knew this. Even though I didn't expect distortion in response, I had every reason to expect some sort of response. What its nature would be I could not dictate. If those incensed by my argument twisted it in anger or indignation, or even by calculation, I cannot complain because I felt innocently surprised by the means to which they resorted. Enter a joust with robust weapons and robust weapons will be used against you.

Why then did I make a contentious argument, knowing full well that it would evoke contention? I compared Holocaust denialism and AIDS denialism because I believed that the comparison between them was valid and true. And illuminating and important. I still do.

More significantly, I made the comparison because I thought it was timely and vital that it be made. It is widely acknowledged that denial of the Nazi Holocaust lacks intellectual or moral respectability. But somehow – as shown in the coverage first the London *Sunday Times* and then the *Spectator* have accorded it – AIDS denialism in its different guises seems to have retained some semblance of intellectual respectability. Perhaps this is because many people still feel genuine uncertainty – or still want to feel uncertainty – about whether an epidemic of such ghastly proportions can really be inflicting suffering and death on such a massive scale in Africa. Perhaps ordinary psychological 'denial' makes some people tolerant of dogmatic denialism.

It was this tolerance that my comparison between the quasi-rationalist methods and the conspiratorialist wellsprings of AIDS denialism and Nazi Holocaust denialism was designed to unsettle. The valid comparison would show, I hoped, that the two forms of knowledge refutation were equally reprehensible morally, and equally discreditable intellectually.

What was more, AIDS denialists were openly and repeatedly boasting that they had secured the ear of President Mbeki. They were a discredited band, but they vaunted their influence. In a country where their legacy of denialist thinking seemed still to be denying the sick and the dying some, or even any, form of public commitment to antiretroviral provision as part of a wider response to their condition, I wanted to challenge the authority and respectability of their doctrines. This I thought was important to establish.

For this I take responsibility.

But I take responsibility also for something more. My interventions on AIDS have explored the limits of judicial participation in current political debate. In many jurisdictions this is a hotly debated issue. In the United States, some judges have held that they are entitled to take part in debates on current political issues. They have invoked their free speech rights in doing so. To prevent them from speaking out about politics, they have argued, is an infringement of their freedom of expression.

I have never shared this view of the judge's role. My view is that judicial office requires those assuming it to accept some limitation on how openly and fully they can participate in public debate on contentious current political issues.

In South Africa and in comparable legal systems such as in England, Scotland and Australia, this is the view most lawyers and judges take. And I think rightly. The justice minister invoked this general principle when he attacked me. He was reported to have complained at a media briefing in Parliament on the day of his attack that 'some judges' issued 'controversial political statements from behind the skirts of their judicial robes'. He appeared to have had my AIDS statements in mind. After repeating the allegation that I called the government's policies on HIV/AIDS and the provision of antiretrovirals 'Hitlerian', he was quoted as saying: 'We must be very careful what we say if we want to preserve the independence of the judiciary . . . and to make sure people respect it.'

The minister was correct to emphasise that care is necessary. I certainly took care in what I said, and how I said it. The question is: was the content of what I said justified? And should I have been the one to say it?

Generally judges should not speak out on current political controversies. There is more than one reason why it is not wise for them to do so. For one thing, the controversial matters on which they may speak out in the political arena may arrive in their courtrooms in the form of legal disputes. If they have committed themselves to a view on one side of the issue, it would not be proper for them to hear the case.

It is for this reason that I have made it plain that I will not sit in a matter involving access to treatment – against a drug company or the government. My public stand as a person with AIDS who owes my own life to the benefit of treatment is that everyone should have a right to life through access to antiretroviral treatment. So strongly and clearly have I expressed this view that my stand has, I believe, disabled me in my judicial capacity from considering with the necessary dispassion legal questions that may arise in this context.

If a question concerning treatment access for persons living with AIDS, whether involving government or corporations, comes to the Supreme Court of Appeal, and the president of our court by oversight assigns me to the case, I will recuse myself.

Such judicial disqualifications are generally undesirable. If judges participate wholesale in public debates on contentious topics that could reach the courtroom, they will have to recuse themselves wholesale from hearing cases. And it is obviously not helpful to have whole sections of a bench of judges disqualified by previous public statement from sitting in important cases. So unless there is compelling justification, the less judges say about vexed current issues, the better.

A second reason is the integrity of the judiciary as a whole. It has an important constitutional role, one that is distinct from government. Government's role is to decide on policy and to carry it into execution. The judiciary's role from time to time is to decide disputes that may arise from implementation of government policy. If judges freely vent their views on current political issues, the impartiality and dispassion of the judiciary as a whole – as the minister rightly suggested – may become suspect. So unless there is compelling justification, the less judges say the better.

A third reason is comity. In a well-functioning constitutional state it is important that there be civility and respect between government and the judiciary. If there should be strain between judges and government, it should be for good reason. Sometimes government's laws or orders or policies have to be overturned on legal grounds. The credit balance in the relationship should be carefully nurtured for use on these occasions. It should not be squandered in unnecessary public ventilation of judges' private views on contentious political issues. Again, unless there is compelling justification, the less judges say the better.

These considerations suggest that judges must think long and hard and carefully before they participate in contentious political debate. That is the principle. But the principle is not inviolate. Judges may be compelled by their personal position, by high dictates of conscience, or by the moral demands of a particular situation, to speak out clearly and forcefully on matters of current controversy. This exception applied, I believe, when I spoke out on dogmatic AIDS denialism.

Everyone now agrees that apartheid was a contentious political issue on which judges should have made their voices heard. As a young practitioner in the courts, I stringently criticised judges holding office under apartheid for their self-seeking and comfortable silence on outrages against justice that were being perpetrated through the legal system. It was one of these attacks that earned me the disfavour of Minister Maduna's predecessor in the justice ministry (Chapter One).

The Truth and Reconciliation Commission (TRC) – South Africa's mighty national effort, in the years following our transition to democracy, to induce the perpetrators of apartheid to own their wrongs, and to find the beginning of a semblance of justice for their victims – pronounced itself clearly on this. It found that 'both the judiciary and the magistracy as well as the organised legal profession were locked into an overwhelmingly passive mindset which characterised the judgments of the bench in the face of injustices of apartheid, and the reaction of the professions to such injustices.'

Not only should lawyers have spoken out against the injustices of apartheid, it said. Judges, the TRC found, should have done so too:

'During the period 1960 to 1990, the judiciary and the magistracy and the organised legal profession collaborated, largely by omission, silence and inaction, in the legislative and executive pursuit of injustice.' This, surely, was a reminder to the country's post-democracy judiciary not to collaborate, by 'omission, silence and inaction', in injustice.

Yet none of this tells us when judges should speak out. There is after all an important difference between apartheid and the present. Judges now hold office under a democratic constitution. There are many mechanisms in our new society to hold the legislature and the executive accountable. Does this lessen the duty resting upon judges to avoid 'omission, silence and inaction' in the face of injustice?

Not always. In May 2000, Chief Justice Arthur Chaskalson delivered the Bram Fischer Memorial Lecture, honouring a brave Afrikaner lawyer who allied himself (through the Communist Party) with the black majority's struggle for freedom and justice. He died while serving a life term for treason against the apartheid state. In paying tribute to Fischer, Chaskalson sounded a telling warning against the direction he considered too many in South African society were taking:

'The constitution offers a vision of the future. A society in which there will be social justice and respect for human rights, a society in which the basic needs of all our people will be met, in which we will live together in harmony, showing respect and concern for one another. We are capable of realising this vision but in danger of not doing so. We seem temporarily to have lost our way. Too many of us are concerned about what we can get from the new society, too few with what is needed for the realisation of the goals of the constitution. What is lacking is the energy, the commitment and the sense of community that was harnessed in the struggle for freedom.'

Chaskalson's words were not a merely anodyne injunction to holiness and virtue. They seemed to have a pointed focus on governmental policies whose redistributive effects were accused of empowering and enriching a small elite. The newspapers reported his comments as implying criticism of the government policies.

Chaskalson, perhaps because of his stature and the guarded nature of his comments, drew no criticism for his intervention.

In early 2001, as the constitutional crisis in Zimbabwe led to scenes of what appeared to be government-sponsored lawlessness in the Zimbabwean courts, and as Chief Justice Anthony Gubbay was coerced into early retirement, the judges of South Africa's two highest courts, the Constitutional Court and the Supreme Court of Appeal, issued a statement warning that the events risked irreversible damage to the rule of law and the credibility of the courts. 'All South African judges,' the heads of the two courts said, 'are concerned when the rule of law is eroded, particularly in a neighbouring country.'

Zimbabwe is a simmering political question which, after AIDS, is perhaps the most contentious area of government policy in democratic South Africa. No one suggested that the judges should not have spoken out on the imperilment of the rule of law in Zimbabwe. Even in a democracy, therefore, there are times when judges must speak out about politically contentious issues. There are times when they must speak out about injustice.

AIDS, similarly, is a highly contentious political issue in our country. But it is contentious only because conventional scientific and medical premises in approaching the epidemic have been disputed. If AIDS denialists had not for a while secured the ear of government, there would have been no fraught overtones in talking about the epidemic and how to deal with it. Saying that people needed treatment would have been as uncontentious as saying that poverty and inequality and racism are wrong. To urge that AIDS be treated as one of the most urgently pressing issues of government, and to say that the epidemic is one of the major moral issues of our time – a test case of how our society responds to moral crisis – would have been uncontroversially obvious.

Given that elementary premises about the causes of AIDS were disputed, and that government's duty to provide treatment was contentious, should I have spoken out so clearly and so controversially? Given the just inhibitions that bind those holding judicial office in a democratic state, I accept that I should not have done so *unless I had compelling justification*. Unless there was profound justification for me to speak out, I accept that I may have erred in discerning the dead hand of denialism in government's policies on AIDS, and in comparing the knowledge system that underlay it to systematic denial of the Nazi Holocaust.

Was there compelling moral justification for me to speak out? I thought so. I still do, though I cannot pretend that I am completely certain about the answer. Part of what makes me uncertain is that I would so like it to have been different. I would so like this controversy never to have taken place.

I am a judge. From the time I started in legal practice, in the dark apartheid days of the early 1980s, I wanted to be a judge. I never thought I would ever hold office as a judge. First, in the unlikely event that I would ever have been offered appointment under apartheid, I would not have accepted it. Later, regardless of the dawn of democracy, I thought I would never hold office because I expected to die from AIDS.

But I did not die of AIDS. I survived to see a democratic transition. I survived to see the inauguration of a visionary and far-sighted constitution, one that not only entrenches existing rights, but also offers the poor and the weak the promise of basic social and economic rights: a framework that offers all South Africans the opportunity for a just society under law.

I survived for President Mandela to appoint me to the High Court under the new constitution. And in October 2000, despite some measure of controversy about my keynote speech at the Durban international AIDS conference, President Mbeki accepted the recommendation of the Judicial Service Commission that I should be appointed to the Supreme Court of Appeal, the country's highest court in non-constitutional matters. (There is some argument that the president is obliged to accept the recommendations of the Commission for High Court and Supreme Court of Appeal appointments; but it is also possible to make the contrary argument: the point is that no one in the president's office sought to make it.)

I love my work as a judge. The intellectual challenges can be exhilarating. And the sense of participating in a transition from a deeply unjust system, enforced through law, to a newly just system, created under a visionary constitution, is rewarding and often inspiring. If AIDS had not happened, if the denialist controversy had not happened, I would have felt blessed in my judicial insulation from contentious political controversy.

But I am not only a judge. I am also living with AIDS. I live in a country in which – on accepted figures – perhaps four or five million people are living with AIDS. I am still the only person holding public office in South Africa who has chosen to make public my HIV status. When the agony of denialism beset our country, I felt I was called to witness. I felt called to account for my survival in a country in which hundreds of thousands were dying unnecessary deaths. I felt called to state the truth about my survival on the very treatment that was being denied to others because of the denialist debate that was taking place. I felt called to speak, and to speak out, and to challenge untruth and obfuscation in the debate about AIDS and its causes and to speak the truth about the proper treatment for AIDS. I did not feel I could or should remain silent.

I felt morally impelled to speak, not merely by knowledge or belief or insight, but by the fact of my survival. This provided that rare justification that is needed for a judge to become involved in political contention. And I felt I would flinch from duty if I remained silent in the face of it.

When I spoke out, the government's commitment to treatment – unexpectedly unveiled in August 2003 – was neither known nor anticipated. That plan has now been announced, and in April 2004 the first treatment sites began to provide the first antiretroviral drugs to poor patients at public hospitals. In his State of the Nation address at the opening of the new Parliament after the second democratic elections of April 2004, President Mbeki announced that one of his government's delivery goals was to have 53 000 people with AIDS on 'treatment' by March 2005. He did not say 'antiretroviral treatment'. He said 'treatment'. But he did say *'treatment'*.

This was a significant and hopeful statement. Perhaps it signalled the end of a dire controversy, and the beginning of hope: the beginning, too, of the mundane, ordinary, vast and indispensable task of saving the lives of nearly five million South Africans who risk death from AIDS unless they have the option of proper care and treatment. Perhaps my speaking out may have played a small part in triggering movement in a situation where for too long action seemed tragically stalled. If that is so, then it must have been right for me, as a person with AIDS, one who is privileged with the luxury of survival when many, many tens of thousands are dying, to speak out.

Given the extent of the crisis, and given my personal experience of the proximity of death from viral infection, and my personal delivery from it through access to care and medication, could I have remained silent? Could I have refrained from speaking while these issues of truth, these issues of entitlement to life and freedom from death, were being determined on our national stage?

My conscience said no. It still does. Whether that was correct will be for a later, more mature, better informed and more objective judgment to determine.

6 | 'We are not the Red Cross' – Patents, profits and death from AIDS
(with *Nathan Geffen*)

It was 9 May 2000, at the start of the wet Western Cape winter. Christopher Moraka was about to give evidence before a legislative committee of the South African Parliament in Cape Town. He came that morning from his home 25 kilometres away in Nyanga, a shanty suburb alongside the busy highway that brings scores of visitors to one of the world's most beautiful cities. What brought Christopher to Parliament was a wonderful chemical substance called fluconazole. It is used to treat candidiasis or thrush. Oesophageal thrush is a painful fungal infestation of the throat. Those who have it find it increasingly difficult to swallow. If not treated, it can be fatal. The fungus's white spores cover the tongue, the palate, the throat, the gullet and eventually the stomach and the whole intestinal system.

As a treatment for thrush, fluconazole works extremely well. Its antifungal agent works by inhibiting what medical scientists call 'fungal synthesis'. Within days most patients recover. The fungal spores disappear from the body. Even in worst cases, the medication needs to be taken for only a fortnight. In addition to its wonderful effects on thrush, fluconazole is also a superb remedy for cryptococcal meningitis. This opportunistic disease affects many AIDS patients in Africa.

I know all this from first-hand experience. When I fell ill with AIDS in October 1997, one of the manifestations that was most distressing to me was oesophageal thrush. My tongue and throat felt furry. They were speckled with what in the mirror looked like grey-white fluff. With horrified revulsion I thought: fungus grows on dead and dying bodies. The unavoidable conclusion was that my body was dying. Physically, my appalled inference was exactly right. My body was dying. And without treatment I would have been dead within 30 to 36 months of the onset of full AIDS.

Symptomatically, my gullet, decked with the furry spores, became hypersensitive to any warm or hot liquid. The spores had spread through my digestive system. I was no longer able to digest food. Like Christopher nearly three years after, I was losing weight and strength.

But I was fortunate. Judges in South Africa have medical insurance, and the insurance covered expensive medication such as fluconazole. So my doctor prescribed it for me. Amidst a host of life-imperilling symptoms, dealing with my thrush was relatively simple. He sat down and wrote out a script and handed it to me. I took it to my pharmacist. Together with the antibiotics that I needed to treat the pneumocystis carinii pneumonia (PCP) that was infecting my lungs, the charges for the antifungal medicine – which at the time were about R120 (or US$20) per dose – were debited to my credit card. In due course the judges' medical insurance scheme repaid me what I had laid out.

So simple: simple for me, and for anyone with access to medical services and available drugs.

The script my doctor wrote out in October 1997 was for fluconazole, manufactured and distributed in the form of a brand-name drug called Diflucan. Pfizer, one of the world's largest pharmaceutical manufacturers, manufactures Diflucan. It worked wonderfully for me. I remember telling my doctor at the time that I believed I could feel its beneficent effects – repelling the spores, cleansing the organisms, opening the cells – within minutes of swallowing the precious capsule. I remember the relief and gratitude I felt at the thought that thrush, at least, was one thing that my body, chemically assisted, would master.

In 2000 Christopher Moraka, too, had oesophageal candidiasis. Badly. One of the last images of him is on a popular television programme, *Beat-It*, that is dedicated to educating the public about AIDS. Interviewed from his bed, Christopher tells of his illness. In a barely audible voice he rasps, 'It's no picnic.' But no one prescribed fluconazole for him. He could not afford it. When Christopher testified before Parliament two and half years after fluconazole had cleared my thrush, Pfizer's branded product Diflucan had come down in price by about one-third. But it still cost over R80 per day. The two-week prescription for Diflucan that Christopher needed, supplied from a private pharmacy, would run to the unimaginable sum of R1 120 – almost as much as the average monthly income of a South African household.

Christopher was unemployed and could clearly not afford to pay Pfizer's prices. He was in any event too sick to be able to work. But he was by no means idle. Some time before, he and his partner Nontsikelelo Zwedala had started a support group for people with HIV at their local clinic. The group they had gathered now numbered more than ten. Both Christopher and Nontsikelelo were members of the Treatment Action Campaign (TAC), a nationwide activist grouping seeking to widen access to AIDS medications. Among the first black people in Cape Town to speak openly about their HIV status, they spent much of their time organising TAC activities in Nyanga township.

Christopher came to tell Parliament's health committee how not being able to afford fluconazole imperilled his life. His testimony had a profound impact. He explained how with the drug, the fungus's attack on his wellbeing could be repelled, and his body could concentrate its remaining energies on defending against other AIDS-related onslaughts. Without it, his agony would increase. His story was stark, and its implications irrefutable.

In theory, fluconazole was supposed to be available in the public healthcare system. But few clinics and hospitals managed to stock it. Even though in 2000 Pfizer charged the government much less than the private-sector price of R80 per dose, the cost of Diflucan was still huge. The result was that patients using public hospitals – as most South Africans must – who were lucky enough to obtain Diflucan were the rare exceptions.

Simply stated, the fact that Christopher could not afford – and that South Africa's public health system could not give him – fluconazole was the direct result of Pfizer's enforcement of its patent rights. In a number of countries, the chemical and medical equivalent of fluconazole was available cheaply. This was because Pfizer had not managed to take out registered patent rights over it everywhere. In those countries, the necessary chemical components could be put together cheaply and efficiently. And they could be made available as a generic form of fluconazole at a cost well within reach of public health systems caring for poor people like Christopher.

This is what Christopher explained to the special hearing of the parliamentary committee on medicine pricing that morning in May 2000. To underestimate his courage in doing so would be wrong. A few seats to Christopher's right sat representatives of the pharmaceutical industry – well-suited professional public relations experts with a job to do. In front of him sat members of the committee – public representatives whose task was to scrutinise the evidence of those who come to testify. Outside the committee chamber, tea and crustless miniature sandwiches were being served. But neither tea nor bread, however served, were of much use to Christopher. He was desperately ill. He was also addressing the committee in his second language. No one of them shared his Nyanga living circumstances, though to some of the committee members they were by no means unfamiliar.

But Christopher persisted. For him, this was about life and death – his life, and his death, and that of many thousands of others. For him his testimony offered an opportunity to hold Pfizer accountable for denying him access to a life-saving medical substance that should have been available to him.

'Denying him access'? 'Should have been available'? Is that not extreme? No. Poor people are denied access to life-saving medications because of patent rights every day across the world. The daily consequence is suffering and death. This should not be so.

A few short months after testifying in Parliament Christopher was dead. His immune system was devastated. Weakened by the systemic thrush, he had developed a number of other opportunistic infections. His oesophageal candidiasis had become so grave that he could not eat at all, and the pain that crippled his digestion and eating had become intolerable. He died on 27 July 2000. He was buried in an emotional ceremony on 5 August 2000. He was not yet 44.

Christopher Moraka's death focused attention on the unjust application of patent laws in poorer countries which cannot afford to pay high prices for patent medicines, but are prohibited from manufacturing or accessing much cheaper alternatives.

Patents arose in the fulsome flowering of arts and intellect and political debate that occurred in fourteenth and fifteenth century Italy. A patent is a governmentally enforced license conferring an exclusive right for a fixed period on an individual or body to make, use or sell an invention. Mechanisms akin to patents have probably existed since civilisation began. Unless originators of new ideas, particularly ones that made living easier or better, are inclined to selfless public service – and some are – they have little incentive to exploit and disseminate their ideas. So rewards for innovation are good and necessary, and humans may well have established them early in our social history.

But the formal legal concept of granting exclusive rights to market and sell a product for a period of time probably dates back to 1421, when the Republic of Florence granted a patent to an individual for an invention. Just more than half a century later, in 1474, Venice enacted the oldest written patent law.

Britain has the richest history of patents. The Patent Office of England proudly affirms that Britain has 'the longest continuous patent tradition in the world'. The current debates about the advantages and disadvantages of patents were familiar to thinkers in sixteenth and seventeenth century England. Queen Elizabeth I granted monopoly rights to industries new to England. Those wanting to start businesses in competition opposed the system. In 1623, the Statute of Monopolies outlawed the grant of exclusive rights. But there was one exception – for inventions: inventors were granted exclusive rights for fourteen years.

Patents on new inventions are now granted for a minimum of twenty years in Europe and South Africa. In the United States the term is twenty-five years. When a medicine is patented, the patent-holder has exclusive rights to market, sell or license the drug as it chooses.

Pfizer filed in the United States for patent protection for fluconazole on 1 June 1982. Its patent was approved on 13 September 1983, and will expire on 3 July 2005. During this period, in every country where Pfizer has registered patent protection for fluconazole, it alone is entitled to exploit it commercially. This led to higher prices for patent Diflucan. It had to. Economics is not like physics; it has no immutable laws. But one law comes close to predictability. It is the law that monopolies drive prices higher. In Thailand there was competition between multiple companies selling fluconazole. In South Africa and most other developing and developed countries, only Pfizer could sell it. This meant much higher prices. Conversely, competition brings prices down – also in the case of essential medications.

Pfizer registered fluconazole in South Africa. But it did not acquire patent protection in Thailand, or in other Asian countries. This led to a dramatic sequel to the death of Christopher Moraka.

Christopher Moraka's death, and the stark courage of his testimony, spurred the TAC to mount a campaign to persuade South African patent-holder Pfizer to reduce the price of fluconazole. Mark Heywood, head of the University of the Witwatersrand's AIDS Law Project, started negotiating with Pfizer on behalf of the campaigners. Pfizer first made a limited offer – it would donate supplies of its drug to treat AIDS patients suffering from cryptococcal meningitis. But by October 2000 no progress toward the donation seemed to have been made.

Pfizer did not want to loosen its hold on its exclusive South African rights to fluconazole. And it did not want to reduce the price at which it was being marketed in South Africa. The market for fluconazole in South Africa was too lucrative. In addition, its executives might have been concerned about the impact that any concessions they made to South African treatment campaigners might have on their position elsewhere in the world.

While this impasse was developing, the TAC was planning its first civil disobedience campaign. It was named for Christopher Moraka. One August evening in 2000, not long after his death, about five Cape Town treatment activists met at the home of a TAC member, Deena Bosch. They outlined a bold campaign that would garner the organisation both plaudits and notoriety.

As a judge holding office under South Africa's constitution, I had sworn an oath 'to uphold and protect the Constitution and the human rights entrenched in it, and [to] administer justice to all persons alike without fear, favour or prejudice, in accordance with the Constitution and the law'. Although I feel passionate about making treatment available to poor people, I could not and would not have any part in conceiving or planning a campaign to defy the laws of South Africa, including the patent laws. As important, I could not and would not lend my support, overtly or tacitly, to any such campaign. My friends in the treatment access movement knew this and respected my position. So I read of their activities as other South Africans did, in the media, which closely followed the dramatic events that ensued.

The defiance campaign demonstrated the TAC's uncompromising determination to increase access to life-saving medicines for poor people. The group decided to consider importing generic fluconazole into South Africa in defiance of Pfizer's patent rights. Generic medications are manufactured according to the patented specifications – but they are not marketed or sold under a brand name. The group wanted to get stocks of fluconazole abroad – not manufactured by Pfizer – and import them for distribution in South Africa in breach of Pfizer's exclusive marketing rights in this country.

The group gave careful consideration to the fluconazole that a number of generic companies produced. The generic fluconazole had to be shown convincingly to be safe, effective and of high quality. Eventually they settled on a product called Biozole. A Thai company, Biolab, manufactured it. A study by medical experts, checked and double-checked by their peers, showed that Biozole was the exact equivalent of Pfizer's Diflucan. What was more, the World Health Organisation had found that Biolab's manufacturing plant met industry standards. Biozole was moreover used quite widely across Asia. And the Paris-based 1999 Nobel prize-winning doctors' organisation, Médecins Sans Frontières – with whom the TAC had developed a close working relationship – recommended it for use.

Travel arrangements were made for Zackie Achmat to travel to Thailand. There he would meet the head of Biolab and determine if importing a large stock of Biozole – for use by people dying unnecessarily from oesophageal thrush, and from cryptococcal meningitis, as Christopher Moraka did – would be practical. Jack Lewis, Zackie's former lover, now housemate and a professional film-maker, went with him to document the trip.

On 17 October 2000, Achmat and Lewis returned to South Africa.

They walked through customs at Johannesburg International Airport. Inside Achmat's bag were 3 000 capsules of Biolab-manufactured fluconazole. Each capsule had cost Achmat a mere two South African rands (about 25 US cents at the time). This was one-fortieth of the price that Pfizer charged in the private sector – which was R80 per capsule. And it was fourteen times less than what Pfizer was charging the South African government for its version of the drug – which was no safer, no more effective and no more useful than the cheaper version.

The next day the TAC held a press conference where it announced the Christopher Moraka Defiance Campaign. The name drew on South Africa's rich history of challenges to apartheid, when black people and some white liberals and socialists united in the 1950s to oppose the demeaning 'pass laws' that required blacks in urban areas to have stamped permission for their presence, and that forced others out of the cities, under great suffering and systematised humiliation, into impoverished rural areas.

For days, the exploit occupied local media attention; it also received extensive international coverage. Debates were organised between Achmat and representatives of the pharmaceutical industry. The South African public were informed about the mathematics of pricing, the effect of patent laws, and the disparities in access to medicine. They also learned about the colossal profits that pharmaceutical companies earn: in 1999, the year before Christopher testified, and died, fluconazole generated more than US$1.002 billion for Pfizer in worldwide turnover.

At the time, the TAC, founded just two years before, was a fledgling organisation, running on a shoestring budget. It seldom operated with legal advice, which could be expensive to obtain. As a result, those planning the campaign made a serious mistake. They aimed their civil infraction at Pfizer. In doing so, they focused solely on Pfizer's patent rights. They thought that Achmat's action would break only patent laws and thus that only Pfizer would be able to take legal reprisals against him.

This proved to be wrong. The activists' plans overlooked the fact that Achmat had also breached South Africa's importation laws regarding unregistered medicines. Under the Medicines Act, illegal importation of drugs can carry a jail sentence of as long as ten years. The police arrived at the Achmat/Lewis home in Muizenberg, Cape Town, a few days after the media conference to seize the contraband shipment of fluconazole.

But the public temper seemed to favour Achmat, and charges were never pressed. The Medicines Control Council – the statutory body that regulates drug quality and importation – gave an HIV specialist working with TAC, Dr Steve Andrews, a special exemption, which permitted him to continue importing Biozole at the knock-down Asian prices. The TAC continues to import fluconazole. With Médecins Sans Frontières, it also began to import antiretroviral medications in breach of patent. But this time it ensured that its earlier error was not repeated.

In changing public understanding and perception, the defiance campaign seemed to have achieved a great deal. The activists' challenge placed Pfizer in an extremely difficult public position. The facts were stark, and their implications for the debate about patent protection, drug pricing and the unnecessary deaths of poor people seemed even starker. The price difference between Biolab-manufactured Biozole and Pfizer's Diflucan was undeniably staggering. It was inflicting hideous suffering – and claiming lives – in South Africa. Nothing in manufacturing costs, marketing expenses or research and development investment could justify it.

What the TAC wanted was that Pfizer should immediately reduce the price of Diflucan. Alternatively, it wanted Pfizer to relax its patent rights to allow another manufacturer to produce a generic version of the product in South Africa. These demands Pfizer rejected. But after the dramatic episode of the contraband Biozole it agreed to donate Diflucan in large quantities for use in South Africa's public health facilities. This was a significant step, and a wise, public-spirited corporate move. Pfizer's decision benefited also other poor countries: currently it provides its own Diflucan free of charge at 987 sites in twenty-five countries that the epidemic has hit hardest.

The success of the Christopher Moraka campaign spread beyond the fluconazole issue. The inequality in access to medicine between the well off and the almost destitute was now in public view. A problem affecting the life and health of millions of third-world citizens was now discussed in many countries, dramatically highlighted by Christopher Moraka's death. Other major pharmaceutical companies have followed with donations of drugs, and some supply lower-cost drugs for countries worst affected by AIDS.

Today, because of Pfizer's donation, over four hundred of South Africa's three thousand public health facilities receive regular deliveries of fluconazole. The majority of facilities can still not obtain the medicine. So the situation is still far from satisfactory. But many more poor people get the drug. In simple practical terms, many lives are saved. And much suffering and discomfort is avoided. Without the Christopher Moraka defiance campaign this would not have happened.

But larger questions about patent enforcement remain. In the last two decades, there has been growing pressure on developing countries to implement patent legislation. This has led to a series of international agreements culminating in the World Trade Organisation's (WTO) Trade Related Aspects of Intellectual Property Rights (TRIPS) Agreement. Given that the brunt of the AIDS epidemic is affecting developing countries, it is the enforcement of exclusive patent rights on life-saving medicines that has caused the most heated global debate.

The TRIPS agreement was signed in Marrakesh on 15 April 1994. It obliges countries party to the WTO (now numbering more than 140) progressively to implement minimum standards of protection for intellectual property. Most developed countries had already implemented patent protection that complied with TRIPS, or they needed to make only slight legislative modifications.

With many developing countries the position is very different. They have to introduce substantial changes. The deadline for complying with TRIPS depends on whether a country is 'developing' (1 January 2000) or 'least-developed' (1 January 2006). Disputes about what TRIPS required of developing countries led to critical negotiations between government ministers in Qatar in November 2001. After an exhausting meeting, a joint statement was issued – the 'Doha Declaration'. This extended the period for least-developed countries to conform to TRIPS to 2016. Further extensions thereafter are possible.

Developing countries had obtained a breathing space before being subjected to the rigorous requirement of uniform patent laws.

Under its present rules, TRIPS has a mechanism that allows governments under certain circumstances including a public emergency such as AIDS to force patent-holders to allow competition. This allows governments or the courts to issue a license to produce the patented product even without the permission of the patent-holder. This is called a compulsory license. Under this power, a pharmaceutical company can be compelled to license a competitor to produce, import and sell generic versions of a patented medicine. The Doha Agreement also made a general statement of great importance in the debate about intellectual property. It affirmed that 'the TRIPS Agreement should be interpreted and implemented so as to protect public health and promote access to medicines for all'. This enshrines the principle the World Health Organisation publicly advocated and advanced – the right of WTO members to make full use of the safeguard provisions of the TRIPS Agreement to protect public health and enhance access to medicines.

Legally, a patent on a medicine is similar (though not identical) to a patent on a new high-tech component of a household appliance. And the legal protections associated with patents on drugs that are not necessary to save lives (such as Viagra) are also similar, though not identical, to those for a patent on a life-saving antiretroviral (such as AZT).

Critics of the current patenting system for medicines acknowledge that innovation should be rewarded. There can be little question that companies that develop new drugs should be rewarded, and that they should be encouraged to innovate. They should also be compensated for the cost as well as the risk of their research and development.

But the legal concepts and mechanisms by which patent rights are granted and enforced are rightly the subject of intense contestation. The law makes a patent, which is the exclusive right to use knowledge, a form of property – 'intellectual property'. Yet in fundamental respects 'intellectual property' differs from other forms of property that enjoy legal protection. So it is misleading to equate patent rights with traditional forms of property such as land. For one thing, land and other resources are limited. And vulnerable: most movable forms of property can be destroyed. Knowledge by contrast is unlimited in time and extent – it can be replicated indefinitely and cannot be destroyed.

For one person to have a finite resource such as food or shelter or land another must not have it. This exclusivity of possession requires implied or express force – in order to keep others out. But knowledge is entirely different. Once an idea is publicly known, no force is needed to appropriate it. It is intangible. And it is replicable. So ideas are susceptible to non-coercive appropriation through copying.

It is only by creating exclusive property rights in knowledge – and thus creating scarcity – that knowledge is transformed into a limited resource. Knowledge can command a price only once it is accorded commodity status. But unlike other forms of property, scarcity is not physical – it is created by the laws that the state enacts. So patent rights have less moral force than other forms of property rights.

Is it justified to challenge and even break patents in the fight for access to essential medicines to treat HIV/AIDS? The answer treatment activists give draws on the special legal nature of patent rights. Patents are created for the public benefit: the theory is that the state grants a patentee a limited statutory monopoly so as to encourage inventors to put their inventions into practice (because by doing so they obtain the financial rewards their inventive efforts warrant).

But current advocates of extended enforcement of patent rights do not always emphasise the benefit to the public – which is an essential part of the theory. So the important question in access to AIDS medications is not whether there should be patent protection – on this everyone agrees – but whether patent protection has become too great. And the question is whether the profits patents earn for their inventors are not disproportionately vast, given the public benefit that underlies the system, and the terrible suffering and death that results from too-stringent protection.

The pharmaceutical industry is not only defensive of its own 'turf', but aggressive about expanding to potential 'turf' throughout the world. In an extraordinary incident in 2000, British pharmaceutical giant Glaxo Wellcome PLC tried to stop an Indian manufacturer of generic drugs, Cipla, from distributing a generic version of a combination drug (AZT and Lamivudine, which Glaxo Wellcome markets as 'Combivir') in Ghana. It seems that Glaxo Wellcome did this even though it did not have a patent on this medicine in Ghana.

Yet, puzzlingly, even though the current international system – especially after the Doha Declaration of November 2001 – grants developing countries leeway, at present they are not fully exploiting it. For instance, they have not been assiduous in issuing compulsory licenses under the exemption that TRIPS grants for emergencies. Part of the problem has been huge pressure against compulsory licenses from the pharmaceutical industry and from the United States and European governments.

In southern Africa, Mozambique and Zimbabwe have issued compulsory licenses for antiretrovirals. But it is not clear that the medicines for which Mozambique issued the licenses were in fact patented. And Zimbabwe's health system, together with its legal system, has been severely damaged by its government's perilous assault upon the rule of law in recent years. This renders the license nearly meaningless within Zimbabwe and as an example for the world. Malaysia too has issued a compulsory license. But the royalty fee details for the patent-holder are tied up in a court battle. So the license has not yet been implemented. This represents desperately slow progress in utilising a public health emergency exception to patent enforcement that everyone acknowledges is now allowed by international law.

The pharmaceutical industry has eloquent and resourceful defenders. They have to be, for there is a great deal (including a great deal of money) at stake. President George W Bush's Trade Representative, Robert Zoellick, is a redoubtable defender of the current system, as is (with some ambivalences) his European Union counterpart, Pascal Lamy. Some non-governmental organisations (such as Africa Fighting Malaria and the Inter-region Economic Network) join them in propounding a range of arguments in favour of stronger patent protection and in opposing compulsory licenses.

They urge persuasively that drug companies must recoup their research and development costs so as to have an incentive to continue to develop new life-saving medicines. Other arguments are less plausible – such as that encouraging development requires even more stringent protections; and that international enforcement of patents adds no additional obstacles to those that poverty already imposes in denying poor people access to life-saving drugs.

It is correct that research and development is a massive cost in evolving new medicines. A company may put millions, perhaps hundreds of millions – even billions – into developing a new cure or treatment that never eventuates. But even such risk of failure does not justify excessive patent protection.

Nor will compulsory licenses by poor countries that have to deal with millions of AIDS deaths impede innovation. The research and development of many antiretrovirals such as AZT, ddi, ddC, d4T and abacavir received significant public support from United States taxpayer money. These drugs were developed at public institutions, such as universities and federal disease and research institutes. The same applies to many other essential medicines.

Besides, drug companies receive huge tax concessions to help them with research and development. This is a form of government subsidy which should be factored in when the sums drug companies say they spend on research and development are considered.

In 1988, the US National Cancer Institute estimated that it spent on average between US$2.3 and 6 million to research and develop a new drug through to the end of Phase III trials. ('Phase III' is the final testing stage where a new drug is tested for efficacy in humans.) This estimate forms a basis, updated from 1988, to compare drug company costs. The 'opportunity costs' of capital (what the company could have earned by investing the money elsewhere), and the risks drug companies run in respect of failed drug developments, must also be added to the equation.

Drug companies claim that it costs about US$800 million to develop a new drug. .They do not however disclose publicly the information that would verify this claim, which was calculated on the basis of privileged information that was disclosed to researchers at Tufts University – but to no others. The $800 million claim is therefore disputed and must be treated with some scepticism. But even assuming the claim is true, there is something more to the whole debate about research and development. The drug companies argue that they need huge profits to develop new drugs. But the profits drug companies earn are already colossal. The 'Fortune 500' and 'Fortune 1000' are *Fortune* magazine's listings of the top United States corporations. In 2002, the pharmaceutical industry had, just behind banking and savings, the highest proportion of profit in relation to sales (return on revenue) in the Fortune 1000 listing. This is perhaps the most telling way of measuring profitability, because it allows us to compare the performance of corporations of all sizes. High returns on revenue for commodities – such as life-saving drugs – provide evidence that mark-ups are massive.

In 2002, the returns for the pharmaceutical companies in the Fortune 500 were on average 17 per cent. This was more than five times the median for all Fortune 500 companies. United Kingdom based Glaxo Wellcome's return on revenue in 2002 was 31 per cent. This was ten times the median average for the same companies (3.1 per cent) – and double that for the nineteen pharmaceutical companies in the Fortune 1000 (16 per cent). The return on revenue in 2002 for Merck was 14 per cent – more than four times the Fortune 500 median average. Merck's revenues in 2002 were US$51 billion – more than the annual revenue of the government of the Republic of South Africa.

These incontestable facts are suggestive. They indicate that despite the alleged burden of research and development costs, pharmaceutical companies are quite phenomenally profitable. It is profits of this order that makes the debate about illness and death in Africa so heart-rending.

Africa south of the Sahara accounts for just over one per cent of worldwide pharmaceutical company sales. Most of these sales are in South Africa, which has Africa's largest and most flourishing economy. To allow other African countries to grant compulsory licenses to manufacturers to produce essential medications would have little impact on pharmaceutical profits.

In any event, compulsory licenses usually yield royalty payments. With a large and expanding market for antiretroviral medicines in southern Africa – itself created by the granting of compulsory licenses – a five per cent royalty on every generic drug sold would eventually yield a reasonable risk-free return for patent-holders.

What the current system of patent enforcement fails to do is to provide incentives to drug companies to spend money on under-researched diseases of the developing world, instead of inessential 'luxury' medicines – for impotence, or hair loss – for affluent first-world residents.

Some suggest that patent protection is a universal necessity and a universal good. They argue that patents are essential for any society to develop, and that countries that implement intellectual property protection are rewarded with success and economic development, and that without patent protection these advantages remain elusive. Arguing this way confuses correlation with cause. Many societies have developed quickly even though they have not respected patents (Malaysia, Thailand, and now also China are examples). Conversely, South Africa protects patents as rigidly as the developed world – yet for many decades it has hardly surpassed its developing world competitors in growth and development.

A recent scholarly study suggests that in nineteenth century Switzerland, Denmark and the Netherlands, it was the absence of patent protection that spurred some of the best inventions. During the industrial revolution, the United States – which now wants to enforce undifferentiated worldwide intellectual property protection – certainly benefited from copying unprotected English inventions.

Until the TRIPS agreement made worldwide patent protection an apparently imperative priority, patents tended to be introduced only when a country's development had reached the point where enough influential inventors lobbied for it. But there is no convincing proof that patent protection is a necessary corollary of development. Countries like India and China have a competitive edge in mass-producing raw materials for pharmaceutical products. Their comparative advantage is not linked to their level of patent protection, but to their ability to copy more cheaply than other countries. More developed countries have more skilled (and usually more expensive) labour. Their advantage lies in trying to enforce patent law globally to prevent such copying. While this battle rages, poor people in Africa, like Christopher Moraka, suffer unnecessarily, and die avoidable deaths.

The least persuasive argument made by proponents of uniform patent enforcement is that what restricts access to life-saving medications in poor countries is poverty, and not patents. Of course poor people in poor countries do not have money to buy drugs. That is their underlying condition. But over-rigid patent enforcement further lifts the price of these drugs out of their reach and that of their governments, who might otherwise be able to supply them.

And no one suggests that deaths from AIDS in poor countries are caused *only* by excessive patent protection. Resolving the patent issue is necessary for reducing medicine prices. But it is clearly not sufficient. Although Zimbabwe has issued compulsory licenses for the production and importation of generic medicines, its health system is in parlous shape. Without good governance, respect for the rule of law, and a well-functioning economy, compulsory licenses on antiretrovirals may amount to little more than hollow populism.

Despite all these obvious problems, one of the main reasons many of the drugs remain too expensive for poor people and poor governments is that they are protected by patents – and sold at monopoly prices. Patents create additional obstacles that deny poor people access to treatment.

It is true that drugs, especially antiretrovirals, have come down hugely in price over the last six years. One of the reasons has been the monumental struggle treatment activists have fought to bring down the cost of antiretrovirals. This has resulted in closer matches between the cost of generic antiretrovirals and patented antiretrovirals.

When I started on triple combination therapy in November 1997, after I became very sick with AIDS, my doctor put me on D4T or Zerit (an AZT-type drug), Lamivudine (marketed as 3TC) plus a protease inhibitor called Norvir. A four-week supply of these three drugs cost me nearly R4 000. Even on a judge's salary, this was a staggering monthly cost. At the time, as mentioned earlier, the judges' medical insurance did not cover antiretrovirals. Because of the crippling cost, though also to a lesser extent because of their continuing side effects, I stopped taking protease inhibitors after about eighteen months. My doctor decided that we should try a third drug in a different class. So I switched to nevirapine, which is a non-nucleoside reverse transcriptase inhibitor (NNRTI). When Glaxo Wellcome (now GlaxoSmithKline) brought out its single-tablet formulation of AZT and 3TC, it was much cheaper.

I have stayed on this regimen – AZT and 3TC in a single tablet, plus nevirapine – for more than four years now. (There was a brief change when my doctor, unnecessarily alarmed at a 'blip' in my viral load pattern, put me onto a different NNRTI – Stocrin.) My current regimen costs only about R700 per month (current United States dollar equivalent is $110). A complete generic regimen is available for approximately R300 to R400 per month. Even these much lower prices are expected to come down more over the next few months. One good generic regimen is now available to the South African government at about R100 per month – an accessible cost that seemed unimaginable just a few years ago.

About six million people in the developing world living with HIV/AIDS need access to treatment now. Of these, less than 8 per cent (some half a million) currently have access to medication. Within the developing world, this ranges from as high as 84 per cent access in Latin America to little more than 2 per cent in Africa. Since more than two-thirds of those with HIV or AIDS live in Africa, this means that at this moment very close to six million poor people are dying of AIDS – unnecessarily, given that the medications to manage their condition exist and can be relatively cheaply produced. The struggle to increase access to life-saving medications to avoid their deaths is far from complete.

Yet there is a developing-world success story in the provision of antiretroviral medications to poor people. Brazil is the world's fifth largest country in both area and population, with over 165 million people. Its per capita gross domestic product is similar to that of South Africa. Like South Africa, it also has a highly unequal income distribution: millions live in poverty, while a minority enjoy affluent living circumstances comparable to those in North America and Western Europe.

Despite its economic constraints, Brazil has implemented a model treatment programme. It dispenses AIDS medications to over 100 000 people. According to Médecins Sans Frontières, the number of deaths from AIDS has decreased by half since the treatment programme was introduced. In consequence, UNAIDS has cited Brazil as an example of *best practice*. The Brazilian government has also offered to transfer knowledge and medicines to other countries severely affected by AIDS.

UNAIDS estimates that about 660 000 Brazilians are living with HIV. As in South Africa, most of these are poor people – though South Africa's figure of four to five million dwarfs that of Brazil. Although the disease is growing among women, twice as many Brazilian men are currently infected. Brazil's policy of providing antiretroviral treatment has been achieved by substantial governmental investment in manufacturing generic medicines.

This policy has had tangible results: between 1996 and 2000, the price of antiretroviral medication dropped on average by 72.5 per cent. The prices of imported drugs also declined – but far less: they dropped by an average of only 9.6 per cent. Over 100 000 Brazilians have been placed on treatment. AIDS deaths in major cities have been reduced by approximately 50 per cent. Needless to say, the quality of life of people with HIV and AIDS has improved significantly.

The Brazilian programme has succeeded because of a vibrant activist community – and also because the Brazilian government has shown the will to make it work. That response has lain beyond only government and non-governmental organisations working in AIDS. The UNAIDS *Best Practices* booklet, *The Brazilian Response to HIV/AIDS*, says that it is 'almost unfair to circumscribe civil society's response to the epidemic to the direct action of the AIDS NGOs'. For almost twenty years, diverse sectors of Brazilian society, including trade unions, philanthropic and religious entities, university research centres and non-governmental organisations have cooperated closely in the struggle against HIV.

It was cooperation of this sort for which the South African Constitutional Court pleaded in July 2002 when it ordered the government to make available antiretroviral medications to enable pregnant mothers with HIV to limit the risk of their babies contracting HIV:

'The magnitude of the HIV/AIDS challenge facing the country calls for a concerted, coordinated and cooperative national effort in which government in each of its three spheres and the panoply of resources and skills of civil society are marshalled, inspired and led. This can be achieved only if there is proper communication, especially by government.' The Court continued: 'We consider it important that all sectors of the community, in particular civil society, should cooperate in the steps taken to achieve this goal [of achieving access to treatment].'

But even with governmental will and national cooperation, access to antiretroviral medications for poor people cannot be regarded as assured. Brazil's own efforts were impeded when in 2001 the United States lodged a complaint with the World Trade Organisation (WTO) about Brazil's intellectual property law of 1996. This statute sought to bring Brazil in line with TRIPS. The US government was dissatisfied with a clause that allowed Brazil to issue compulsory licenses where the patent-holder did not produce the patented product in Brazil, and was unable to show that it was economically or legally unviable for it to do so.

At the WTO, Brazil insisted on its right to introduce this clause. It relied on the argument that TRIPS represented a delicate balance – and that attempts by the US to strengthen the level of patent protection threatened to upset that balance. Brazil even questioned whether the US was trying to undermine the Brazilian AIDS programme. After all, the law had been enacted in 1996 – and the US's belated complaint to the WTO seemed to coincide with international focus on Brazil's AIDS programme as a world best-practice exemplar, and with growing pressure on drug companies to reduce prices.

The real threat the US complaint embodied was its chilling effect. If a Brazilian statute licensing local production generated such emphatic US objections, developing countries seemed to be warned off any notion of exporting compulsorily licensed drugs.

The United States challenge to Brazil's compulsory license provision pushed activists into worldwide solidarity action. This coincided with the response to legal action that some forty pharmaceutical companies took against the South African government for legislation that it enacted in 1997 to reduce medicine prices by allowing parallel imports and by removing certain counterproductive incentives in the drug supply chain. For four years, the legislation was held up and South Africa was placed on a United States list that threatened trade penalties.

The South African government and the pharmaceutical companies seemed deadlocked in the litigation until the Treatment Action Campaign entered the fray. The TAC applied to the Pretoria High Court to be granted amicus ('friend of the court') status and to lodge evidence and arguments in the case. This, as AIDS Law Project head Mark Heywood said, turned a dry legal contest into a matter about human lives. The South African media reported extensively on the case. As protest actions increased, the world's media began to notice too.

On 5 March 2001, demonstrations took place in Brazil, the United States, South Africa, Europe and Asia. The demonstrators' demand was that the pharmaceutical companies withdraw their court challenge to the South African legislation. But they also highlighted the US complaint against Brazil at the WTO. Six weeks later demonstrations in favour of the legislation reached a climax in South Africa when the country's largest trade union grouping, COSATU, joined in with thousands of its members. On 19 April the pharmaceutical manufacturers withdrew their case against the South African government when the parties announced a settlement. Though the government pledged respect for patent rights, the legislation remained intact.

Around the world this was hailed as a victory for AIDS activists and the South African government, as well as for increased access to treatment. The balance of power seemed to have shifted, even if only slightly, in the struggle between people without treatment and the drug companies.

The United States complaint against Brazil was also settled on terms that favoured greater treatment access. The two sides negotiated an agreement that the local working clause would stay, though on condition that Brazil undertook to meet certain US pre-conditions should it decide to invoke the law.

Brazil's success in making antiretroviral treatments available to people with AIDS resulted from political will, drug manufacturing capacity, a history of activism and a substantial World Bank loan. Critical too was the Brazilian government's firm alliance with civil society groupings, which contrasted tragically with the approach of the South African government after 2001. The Brazilian government's relationship with activists has not been entirely free of conflict. But the contrast with South Africa is poignant. In Brazil, there has been a spirit of accommodation, mutual acknowledgement and cooperation.

But there were further factors. Brazil did not patent pharmaceuticals until 1997, when it embarked on TRIPS compliance. This late start meant that manufacturers could produce antiretrovirals generically.

Brazil has not issued a compulsory license, though it has threatened to do so with newer patented medicines. This prospect has brought lower prices. The Brazilian government threatened compulsory licenses in respect of drugs produced by Bristol-Myers Squibb, Roche, Abbot Laboratories and Merck. Its threats led drug companies to agree to reduce prices on some antiretrovirals.

The TAC intervention in 2001 in the pharmaceutical industry court challenge to the South African government is rightly credited with helping preserve the 1997 law. Yet Health Minister Tshabalala-Msimang refrained from acknowledging the TAC's role. And she denied that the court victory had enabled the government to introduce an antiretroviral programme. This set off a long and protracted conflict with the TAC. Even today it tragically lingers.

Thailand also has seen vibrant engagements about patents and access to medicines. In early 2004, after a number of court battles over three years with activist groups, Bristol Myers Squibb (BMS) agreed to return its patent on didanosine (ddi), a commonly used antiretroviral, to the 'people of Thailand'. The agreement was concluded between BMS, the Thai Network of People Living with HIV/AIDS, the AIDS Access Foundation and the Foundation for Consumers at the Central Intellectual Property Rights and International Trade Court. Activists rightly emphasised that the victory resulted from hard work, and did not stem from unheralded corporate benevolence. It was the result of a concerted struggle to improve access to life-saving medication.

In South Africa, activists also challenged BMS over the cost of its two antiretrovirals – didanosine and stavudine. American research institutions hold the patents on these two drugs. They in turn exclusively licensed them to BMS. The battle culminated when BMS agreed to a significant price reduction – both medicines now cost only US$1 per day. It is no exaggeration to say that this has given many thousands more South Africans access to life.

Perhaps the most arresting of the struggles about patent rights involved a complaint a group of AIDS activist organisations and individuals lodged in September 2002 before South Africa's Competition Commission. The first complainant was a woman with AIDS, Hazel Tau. She invoked the commission's powers, under the Competition Act of 1998, which gives it wide investigative authority to censure overpricing, price-fixing and other monopolistic practices.

The complainants were the TAC, the AIDS Consortium (a national umbrella body of AIDS organisations), the trade union federation COSATU, one of their affiliates in the chemical industry, healthcare workers and – most tellingly – people living with HIV/AIDS. The AIDS Law Project at the University of the Witwatersrand represented all the complainants, who charged that United Kingdom-based GlaxoSmithKline (GSK) and Boehringer Ingelheim (BI) were unlawfully fixing excessive prices for antiretroviral medicines. BI is a privately owned group of German pharmaceutical companies that owns the patent rights to nevirapine. It was BI that in 2000 imaginatively offered to donate free supplies of nevirapine to all third-world governments needing it for prevention of mother-to-child transmission of HIV.

The complainants' case was that there was a legally proved connection between the drug companies' excessive prices and the premature, predictable and avoidable deaths of women, men and children living with HIV/AIDS in South Africa. This allegation found dramatic embodiment at the very start of the litigation. On 19 September 2002 the complainants held a media conference in Johannesburg to announce their challenge. At the end of the briefing, Hazel Tau, the first complainant, became severely ill. Her CD4 count (which measures the strength of the immune system) was later measured. It was less than 10. Since an HIV negative person generally enjoys a CD4 count of 500 to 1 500, it was clear that Hazel had almost no immune protection at all.

In her affidavit to the commission, Tau explained how she was diagnosed in 1991. As in my own case, she was tested and informed that she was HIV positive without any pre- or post-test counselling. She was given no information about HIV. She was not even told that HIV was incurable: and was accordingly not too upset. For a short period during 1993 she took AZT singly. Her husband's medical insurance covered the cost of this monotherapy. She stopped taking the medicine when she felt better. This was a common experience of patients in the late-1980s and early 1990s who took AZT alone: for a short time, before the virus finds a way around the antiretroviral properties of the single drug, the patient improves. But soon thereafter any benefit is lost. Antiretroviral monotherapy is now recognised as extremely dangerous.

Then her husband locked her out of their house and later divorced her because she had HIV. She said that this had happened without her 'consent or knowledge': 'I never appeared before a court, never was summoned, but found a paper reflecting that I was divorced from my husband.' (Such a procedure is not legally competent in South Africa, where a divorce defendant must be personally informed of the divorce action by formal service of the divorce papers. The defendant then has an opportunity to resist the action. But in my years as a judge in the Johannesburg High Court I did encounter instances where either by collusion or mistake the court papers were served on the wrong defendant. In addition, forgery of the sheriff's 'return of service' is not impossible.)

Tau further stated that as a result she had lost everything she had, including her house, her clothes and furniture. Of course, this also meant that she no longer qualified for benefits under her husband's medical insurance scheme. By 2002 she was destitute, but she needed antiretroviral treatment again. Her CD4 count had dropped to below 200, and since 2000 she had lost 25 kilograms in weight.

At the time of the complaint she was employed to work on an HIV/AIDS help line. But her earnings were insufficient for her to afford a triple combination of antiretroviral drugs. Three antiretroviral drugs would cost her over R1 000 per month at 2002 prices. She testified that she would however be able to afford a generic combination of antiretrovirals for just less than R400 per month, were it available in South Africa.

Hazel Tau's affidavit makes stark and compelling reading. The complaint led to an extensive investigation by the Competition Commission. On 16 October 2003, the commission announced its findings: it held that GSK and BI had contravened the statute. It found that the companies had abused their dominant positions in their respective antiretroviral markets. The commission found that GSK and BI had engaged in outlawed restrictive practices by denying a competitor access to an essential facility by using excessive pricing, and by engaging in an 'exclusionary act'. The commission therefore found grounds to refer the matter to the Competition Tribunal (a body with judicial powers) for determination.

A favourable finding by the tribunal would have entailed a formal determination that the complaints against the drug companies were justified – a rich prize in activists' eyes. Yet there was a risk that the tribunal would not uphold or would modify the commission's findings. There was also the question of precious time: while legal procedures dragged on, the primary objective – getting cheaper drugs to dying people – was delayed. And even if the competition tribunal upheld the commission's determination, that finding was itself subject to appeal to the Competition Appeal Court. Thereafter an appeal would be made to the Supreme Court of Appeal. If a constitutional issue was involved, a further appeal to the Constitutional Court was in prospect.

Weighing all the risks and potential delays, the TAC decided to enter into settlement negotiations with GSK. Shortly thereafter it also started negotiating with BI. Extensive talks aimed at reaching a settlement were conducted between lawyers representing all sides.

Not all those backing the litigation agreed with this strategy, and painful differences within the activist camp emerged. One of the affidavits for the complainants was James Love of the Washington DC-based Consumer Project on Technology. Love, an expert in the economics of patents, has for many years campaigned redoubtably for compulsory licenses. He reasonably set his hopes on an outcome that would lead to the first compulsory license in South Africa.

But TAC leaders considered that making medicines more affordable as quickly as possible was the first imperative. The organisation feared that, although there was a reasonable chance of an ultimate court victory, it would take years before all the possible appeals were exhausted. In addition, the risk of losing outweighed the much quicker and certain benefits that would arise from the settlement agreements.

On 10 December 2003, the complainants accepted comprehensive settlement agreements that would help ensure access to affordable medicines. In exchange, they withdrew their complaint against the two pharmaceutical companies. The settlement agreements entailed that improved, affordable and sustainable access to life-saving medicines could become a reality.

For the first time, GSK and BI agreed to issue multiple licences on their patented antiretrovirals. GSK agreed to grant licences to four generic companies, while BI agreed to grant licences to three companies, to produce and/or import, sell and distribute the antiretroviral medicines AZT and lamivudine. The royalty fee was pegged at no more than five per cent of net sales. This is a crucial step to ensuring that there is proper competition between generic drug companies. Only with sufficient competition can the prices of antiretrovirals reach their lowest possible point and thus become and remain affordable. Crucially, the agreements also allow licensees to export AZT, lamivudine and nevirapine manufactured in South Africa to all forty-seven sub-Saharan African countries.

Many challenges lie ahead. These are to ensure that suitable generic drug companies are speedily licensed. Their drugs must be registered with urgency. Other multinational pharmaceutical companies must be persuaded to follow the lead of GSK and BI. And, most importantly, the South African government must take full advantage of the agreements when it procures medicines for its public sector treatment programme.

By late 2004, the companies had not yet issued all the voluntary licenses. The TAC continues to pressurise the two companies to meet what it considers to be their obligations. But that a breakthrough had been achieved was incontestable. Wits University's AIDS Law Project won the Department of Trade and Industry Consumer of the Year 2003 Award for its work in representing the complainants.

Hazel Tau's story has a relatively happy ending. After her onset of unwellness at the competition challenge media conference in September 2002, a private doctor who runs a treatment programme for a large South African company organised sponsorship anonymously for her. She has since recovered and is well, her HIV-related illnesses under sound control. In her native tongue, seTswana, her name means 'lion': Hazel Lion.

Stories like those of Hazel Tau and Christopher Moraka have energised and dramatised the public debate about the limits of intellectual property protection and its role in access to treatment and innovation. The AIDS epidemic has radically challenged, and altered, the premises on which the debate about intellectual property protection is conducted.

A decade ago, when the TRIPS agreement was concluded at the WTO, the arguments the pharmaceutical industry advanced were largely unchallenged. Today, the very foundations of TRIPS are subjected to intense debate. The stringency of TRIPS's terms has been ameliorated. And pharmaceutical companies find their domination of developing-world markets challenged by patent disputes, compulsory licenses and sustained protests.

There have been a number of proposals to reconceive the international system of patent protection. Two researchers from the Centre for Economic and Policy Research in Washington DC have produced a study that proposes an alternative research system for pharmaceutical products in which public and not-for-profit funding would play a much greater role.

Nathan Geffen of the Treatment Action Campaign and Jonathan Berger of Wits University's AIDS Law Project have on the basis of current ideas and debate proposed two modifications to the current system: greater transparency on research and development costs, so that a more accurate analysis can be made of the extent to which pharmaceutical prices are too high; and a royalty-based (as opposed to an exclusive market-based) patent system, perhaps with investment from a multinational body for companies that develop highly sought-after drugs for high-mortality and under-researched diseases of the developing world. The current system is vulnerable to charges that it suits neither the United States nor developing world consumers. All pay too much for life and health.

In the battle for public support over ideas and systems, the pharmaceutical companies still have greater lobbying power than the activist groups. In the United States presidential elections of 2000 and 2004, the pharmaceutical industry was a significant donor to both candidates. In the US Congress, it is a highly effective lobby.

But pharmaceutical companies have made significant and in some instances humane concessions to demands for treatment access. Pro-treatment movements are likely to continue their vigilance. An executive vice-president of Pfizer, exasperated by the conflict he had to endure over his company's battle with AIDS activists, told a reporter in April 2001: 'We are not the Red Cross. We are a for-profit company.'

This is true. Drug companies are not charitable concerns. It is not their task to care for Christopher Moraka or Hazel Tau. But perhaps this is the very point activists are making. It is precisely because companies are not charitable institutions and cannot be expected to behave as such that the patent system they rely on must be adapted. The world will be a better place, with less misery and fewer avoidable deaths, when we achieve a system of intellectual property protection that protects consumers as much as it benefits large corporations.

7 | Poor treatment – Justice for poor people

(with *Nathan Geffen*)

When Christopher Moraka died on 27 July 2000 of AIDS-related complications, exacerbated by his untreated thrush, his partner of three years, Nontsikelelo Zwedala, was herself unwell. For months she too had been suffering from disabling AIDS-related illnesses – so much so that she could not accompany Christopher when he went to Parliament to testify in May. At Christopher's funeral on 5 August Nontsikelelo seemed painfully alone. Onlookers must have sensed her grappling with anticipation of her own mortality.

Many who knew her could not help thinking that her death was imminent. They had seen many other deaths, many waning lives and many futile, unmedicated struggles. Yet Nontsikelelo continued to attend every picket, every march and every meeting. At a picket in November 2000, shortly after Christopher's death, outside Cape Town's world-renowned public hospital, Groote Schuur – where in 1967 Professor Christiaan Barnard performed the world's first heart transplant – Nontsikelelo even made a public speech. But her frail voice and shyness made it almost impossible for those attending to hear her. Her CD4 count was below 20 – in effect, her immune system was no longer functioning. Death was only a matter of time.

Like Christopher, Nontsikelelo developed severe candidiasis. She too could not afford fluconazole. In her case, the fungus spread to her epidermis, covering her entire body. Desperately, weighing only about 40 kilograms, she would extend her skeletal hands, showing how the white-flecked spores covered them. She seemed to be gesturing vainly for life.

But those awaiting her death underestimated Nontsikelelo's resolve. She wanted to continue her life and work. She was also devoted to her nine-year-old son, Pikolomzi. In late March 2001, eight months after Christopher's death, and close to the end herself, she managed to find a place on a trial for a new antiretroviral drug. This was her only hope. But within a few weeks, she developed an adverse reaction to one of the drugs. Fortunately however she did not experience virological failure (where the virus runs rampant despite antiretroviral treatment). So there was still hope for her. Her doctors considered that she could safely change to a newer, more effective regimen. So within months, she switched to a combination very similar to my own – D4T (Zerit – an AZT-like drug), plus 3TC (lamivudine) and nevirapine. This is the simplest and (for many) most effective combination of antiretroviral drugs. The South African government can now purchase the combination from a generic producer at about R100 per month..

Since this new combination, Nontsikelelo has not looked back. The drugs have proved effective. They have stopped the virus's activity in her body. Her health has returned, and it has remained with her. In September 2002, just eighteen months after starting combination therapy, Nontsikelelo was well enough to join as a litigant in the monopolies complaints against GlaxoSmithKline and Boehringer Ingelheim before the Competition Commission (described in Chapter Six). She was one of eleven complainants who contended that the companies were charging excessive prices for their antiretroviral products – zidovudine (better known as AZT), lamivudine and nevirapine.

Nontsikelelo was using two of the three drugs, and wanted their prices lowered so that she would no longer be dependent only on the drug trial in which she was participating. In a sworn affidavit she submitted to the commission, she described herself as 'a 31-year-old woman living in Philippi in a squatter camp called Kosovo'. Her reference to the geography of her residence was deliberately significant. Kosovo may be one of the least developed areas in Cape Town. The residents – mostly desperately poor – have named their living environment with fitting irony. There is no road directly to Nontsikelelo's shack. A maze of eroded dirt tracks can with difficulty bring a visitor's vehicle within a short walk of her home.

Few homes in Kosovo have the luxury of an indoor toilet, running water or regular electricity. Millions of South Africans live like this. Tens, perhaps hundreds, of millions of Africans, and possibly a billion people around the world, live in the same way. Many millions of Africans and other poor people elsewhere in the world who have HIV live in such conditions.

The critical question that treatment activists, government officials and public health experts have debated in recent years is whether the complex demands that surviving AIDS on antiretroviral treatment entail can be met in such deprived and difficult living conditions.

It is that question this chapter considers. Nontsikelelo's affidavit provided her own answer to the debate. Her answer was calm and clear and incontrovertible. Though as poor as millions of others living with HIV and AIDS, antiretroviral combination treatment had worked for her. Her affidavit told of her dramatic recovery:

'I was on the last stage of the disease and when I started my medication my CD4 count was only 14 and I had a viral load of 3 million. I am taking nevirapine, d4T and 3TC. I was very scared of the side effects but I don't experience any serious side effects anymore. Anyway I would rather live with the side effects than die of AIDS. The minor side effects I had were always monitored by my doctor and he changed the treatment if necessary. I had a problem of forgetting to take my pills during the first month, but I got used to them and committed myself to adhering since I knew that without them I would certainly die. I take them twice daily and my health is improving.'

That Nontsikelelo's health is improving remains salutatorily true. When I spoke to her after she had blood tests in January 2004, she told me that her CD4 count was over 600 – signifying a more than adequately healthy immune system. Her viral load was undetectable. Practically, her medications were paralysing the virus's activity within her body, enabling her immune system to function effectively again. Her treatment is successful.

Every three months she makes the minibus-taxi trip into town to collect her antiretroviral medications. German pharmaceutical manufacturer Boehringer Ingelheim, with whom Nontsikelelo joined issue in the competition commission challenge, sponsors her drug trial. Without it she like Christopher would be dead. And like many millions of children across central and southern Africa, Pikolomzi (his Xhosa name means 'wing of the home') would be orphaned.

Nontsikelelo's current antiretroviral regimen still presents difficulties. She battles lipodystrophy (the poor distribution of body weight that antiretroviral drugs can cause) – a common side effect of many of the drugs, including D4T. But she has life: a productive, healthy and purposeful life. And she can care for her son. In addition, every week she counsels people with HIV at the Sizophila ('We Will Be Well and Healthy') antiretroviral project in Gugulethu, a neighbourhood adjoining Nyanga. Her personal testimony and extraordinary resolve create hope for others starting treatment. While writing this I spoke with her. One of the roosters she keeps was heartily crowing outside her home. I asked her about her work at Sizophila. 'When I was sick,' she explained, 'I promised to give my life to other people.'

In isiXhosa, the tongue of her birth, 'Nontsikelelo' means 'blessing'.

Nontsikelelo's life and health – and her recovery from near-death – are a rebuke to those who have argued that it is impractical or impossible to introduce antiretroviral treatment for poor Africans who have AIDS. Many arguments have been made that treatment in these settings is not 'sustainable': that Africa lacks the infrastructure necessary for the drugs to be used effectively; that the cost of treating Africans is too high; that efforts should rather be concentrated on prevention. But does implementing large-scale treatment programmes require too much money? And are such interventions too complex for the healthcare infrastructures of poor countries?

The arguments are interwoven. A few years ago there was an accepted orthodoxy amongst healthcare planners and government policy-makers. It was this: cost, infrastructure and the need to concentrate available funds on prevention and awareness campaigns ('saving the uninfected') made talk about treating people living in poverty impractical. Both UNAIDS and the World Health Organisation adopted a somewhat muted approach to large-scale access to treatment. Most governments, supported by public health officials, expressed scepticism about providing treatment en masse to poor people with AIDS. Even some funders who now contribute generously to treatment programmes, including George Soros, were not yet persuaded that large-scale treatment in Africa was feasible.

The last five years have wrought a revolution in these attitudes. The principled actions of treatment activists in Africa, Brazil, Thailand, North America and Western Europe were crucial to achieve this change in position.

In South Africa, the challenge to orthodoxy started with the launch of the Treatment Action Campaign in Johannesburg in December 1998. In North America, the challenge to orthodox approaches to making antiretroviral treatment widely available had its most vivid and newsworthy expression when angry activists protesting against Vice President Al J Gore's drug company lobby connections loudly disrupted the launch of his presidential campaign in June 1999.

Just more than a year later, sixteen thousand kilometres away, 5 000 activists – mostly poor and black – marched before the opening of the international AIDS conference in Durban in July 2000. They demanded acceptance of the same principles – that poverty should not be a barrier to life-saving AIDS treatments.

The voices of these activists resonated across the world. In March 2001 several hundred academics from Harvard University signed the Harvard Consensus Statement. It called for wealthy countries to fund treatment programmes in the developing world, and dismissed scepticism about the practicality and efficacy of such programmes.

Soon thereafter, in June 2001, a special sitting of the United Nations General Assembly (UNGASS) was convened to consider international and governmental responses to the AIDS epidemic. The meeting took place in New York in the changed atmosphere that the Durban conference a year earlier had precipitated. UNGASS gave rise to the creation of a multilateral, independent, international financing mechanism called the Global Fund to Fight AIDS, TB and Malaria (GFATM).

The fund's purpose is to finance projects in the developing world to facilitate prevention, treatment and care for the three infectious diseases that exact the highest death toll in the world. The GFATM is the main financing mechanism for achieving the goal the WHO has set itself – that three million people with AIDS should be on treatment with antiretrovirals by the end of 2005.

Hard, practical experience is vindicating claims by activists that treatment for the developing world's persons with AIDS is not only just, but cost-effective and 'sustainable'. Various programmes amongst very poor people show that lack of infrastructure is no barrier to successful antiretroviral treatment. In Brazil, the government's national treatment programme operates amidst less than ideal healthcare infrastructure and services. And in Haiti, the impassioned and outspoken Harvard medical professor, Paul Farmer, runs a highly successful 'Partners in Health' programme.

In Khayelitsha, Cape Town, and Lusikisiki, Eastern Cape, Médecins Sans Frontières (MSF) has treatment programmes for people living in poverty which function extremely well. There are also fledgling antiretroviral programmes that serve non-affluent communities in Botswana, Cameroon and Thailand.

MSF started its Khayelitsha project in May 2001. Patients receive treatment after careful selection, based on medical criteria such as their CD4 counts and general wellness. Also important is the question whether the patient is willing to take responsibility for his or her own treatment: the project adopts a 'patient-centred adherence approach'. This requires patients to have been punctual for their clinic appointments for three months. They must also have a supportive home environment, and someone to help them with their treatment. In late 2004, MSF had more than 1 700 people living on its Khayelitsha programme.

Results have been heartening. More than four-fifths of patients remain in the programme after eighteen months. Treatment is in most instances successful. It's the usual story. The virus succumbs to antiretroviral treatment. The only difference is that this story is played out in highly unusual social circumstances. But the truth is in fact unsurprising. Poor people's viral loads drop dramatically on receiving treatment – like those of more affluent people – and their virus becomes undetectable in blood tests within a few months. Even less surprising is that poor people – like more affluent people –

are keen to stick to their drug regimen, take their drugs properly and secure maximum benefit from them.

And yet the success of these treatment initiatives has been surprising to many who opposed them. The argument for widening access to treatment in resource-poor settings was not easily won, and it is still not completely over. In 2001, at the height of the campaign for rational approaches to treatment in South Africa, and after the UN General Assembly on AIDS, one of the largest United States foundations focusing on health distributed a special insert with South Africa's mass-circulation Johannesburg *Sunday Times*. Entitled 'Impending Catastrophe Revisited: an update on the HIV/AIDS epidemic in South Africa'. It suggested that life-saving antiretroviral treatment on a mass scale was not feasible. Treatment activists experienced its publication as a disheartening rebuff.

The insert conceded that a 'strong argument' could be made for a programme to provide a short course of treatment to prevent mother-to-child transmission of HIV. But it suggested that antiretrovirals to treat AIDS created too many problems to be realistic: 'Paying the full price of antiretroviral therapy would increase the cost of healthcare by R70 billion in 2010. Even if the price were reduced by 90 per cent, the cost would still increase the health budget by R15 billion.'

This missed the point that antiretroviral treatment would reduce the burden of opportunistic infections on the public healthcare system. Instead, the document seemed to suggest that hospice care (and thus death) – and not treatment and recovery – were the answer to problems of rationing in the health system.

'Impending Catastrophe Revisited' predicted that AIDS deaths in South Africa would rise from 120 000 in 2000 to over 540 000 in 2010. It described the resulting impact on households and women, growth in the number of orphans, pressure on the healthcare system, and negative effects on business because of morbidity and mortality caused by AIDS. Yet it shrank from the obvious conclusion that treating people with HIV, using antiretroviral medicines where necessary, would contribute to alleviating these consequences, thus saving millions of lives.

The document also seemed to advance the damaging and erroneous notion that 'prevention is better rather than cure' in AIDS programmes. This argument has done particular harm in the debate about whether treatment provision to poor people is feasible. In general terms prevention rather than cure is a common and sensible wisdom. Everyone prefers to avoid getting sick rather than enduring the symptoms of disease and the medicines needed to treat it. But once someone does fall ill, it seems objectionable to deny them treatment where it does exist. Yet many who have argued that prevention efforts should be the focus of AIDS interventions in Africa have gone further, implying that those who do get sick should be denied life-saving medications.

The prevention-rather-than-treatment argument has proved resilient. Health-specialist writers have continued to contend in respected professional journals like the *Lancet* that preventing HIV infections is more cost-effective than treating people with AIDS. The cost argument against treatment in most southern African countries was also made in a policy discussion paper that the International Monetary Fund circulated in 2001.

At the most elementary level, the arguments against mass provision of antiretroviral treatments ignore the human claims of those who are dying of AIDS. The morality of such arguments is difficult to defend, since treatment exists for AIDS-related conditions and is available: the only question is whether efforts should be directed toward making it accessible to those who still do not have it.

But from the practical perspectives of public health, of development and even of prevention, the anti-treatment arguments are not convincing.

Professor Nicoli Nattrass, an economist at the University of Cape Town, has shown that to contrast the cost-effectiveness of prevention over treatment – as though a simple dichotomy exists between the two – is wrong-headed. She has warned that economic analysis 'becomes dangerous when decision-making power is ceded to seemingly technical arguments without realising the nature of the implicit social judgements behind them'.

This can happen, Nattrass says, when economists use the 'rhetoric of economic expertise' to intimidate critics and to silence debate. For example, she says, a finance minister could defend a government's restriction on resources for antiretroviral therapy by claiming that increased expenditure would 'threaten to undermine the country's sound economic fundamentals'. Her example has a poignant ring, since this, more or less, is what happened in South Africa during the critical years of government inaction on the epidemic.

Nattrass observes that most people do not understand what 'sound economic fundamentals' means. Invoking such vague rhetoric effectively silences debate. Yet the truth is that government spending decisions are made not only on the basis of 'cost efficacy'. They are also determined – quite rightly – by government's political objectives, as well as by a host of judgments about social preferences and economic behaviour.

Government planners in other words make deliberate choices. They are not ineluctably compelled by abstract economic 'realities'. Those choices can include – or exclude – the critical decision whether to save those dying from AIDS by giving them access to antiretroviral medications.

The point seems obvious. But the rhetoric of 'sound economics' has obfuscated the debate about AIDS treatments in South Africa, and for too long delayed their implementation. In late 2002, after months of formal negotiations between government, business, labour and community sector representatives, government was on the brink of signing an agreement. This would ultimately have committed it to providing antiretroviral treatment in public-sector hospitals. At the last moment, government pulled out of the negotiations. The health minister gave as reasons the cost and the complexity of implementing antiretroviral treatment. It took another eighteen months, and many more deaths, before the cabinet agreed to public provision of treatment.

This deadly delay seemed to have less to do with cost and complexity than with lack of political commitment to the viral theory of AIDS within government's own leadership.

Cost-efficacy and 'sustainability' remain redoubtable questions. In June 2002 the Treatment Action Campaign and the Congress of South African Trade Unions, together with doctors' professional and other health worker groups organised a treatment conference in

Durban. I was invited to speak at the closing ceremony. At the meeting, organisers distributed a paper that rebutted the arguments that treating poor people with AIDS was not 'cost-effective'. This is an elementary point about human rights. It is quite simply unethical and immoral to invest money in preventing new HIV infections while allowing millions who are already infected to die.

Besides, as United States Secretary of State Colin Powell declared in 2001, the death and incapacitation and suffering that the epidemic is causing in sub-Saharan Africa constitutes a security threat to Africa and to the world.

Most analysts now accept the prevention/treatment dichotomy is false and unhelpful in determining options for action. Prevention strategies will be less effective unless treatment forms part of the overall plan. A study in East Africa shows that voluntary counselling and testing is an effective way of changing sexual behaviour. Yet those willing to accept counselling and testing will remain few so long as the testing and counselling process offers them nothing concrete. Treatment is a significant inducement to be tested, and finding one's health restored – as I did in 1997 – is a huge incentive to telling others about HIV and about healthy living.

But in most poor countries infection with HIV is still wrongly regarded as a death sentence. Why get tested if the only 'benefit' is to gain knowledge of one's own premature death – with the added likelihood of discrimination and stigma? By contrast, when treatment is offered as part of a voluntary counselling and testing programme (including a safer-sex discussion and condom provision), there is a real incentive for people who suspect that they may have HIV to come forward.

Ultimately treatment and prevention cannot be separated without sacrificing the quality of both.

A costing study that Nathan Geffen, Nicoli Nattrass and Chris Raubenheimer prepared in 2003 demonstrates that the maximum amount of money the South African government could usefully spend on HIV prevention interventions (such as voluntary counselling and testing, mother-to-child transmission prevention and improved treatment of sexually transmitted infections) is very small in terms of the overall health budget. Once money for all these cheaper prevention programmes is allocated, the only further expenditure on HIV/AIDS that would be cost-effective is for antiretroviral treatment.

The analysis shows that both treatment and prevention could simultaneously be implemented in South Africa over a thirteen-year period – saving millions of lives – without imposing unmanageable budget constraints.

Health economists making the contrary argument compare the HIV epidemic in the developing world to the necessity of 'triage' during wartime. 'Triage' describes the desperate situation where battlefield doctors and off-field healthcare personnel must in crisis-time assign degrees of urgency to soldiers' and civilians' wounds or illnesses to decide in what order to treat them. 'Now for perhaps the first time in history,' a group of writers recently intoned in a medical journal, 'we must decide whether economic reality will permit an informed debate about rationing that could result in millions of patients receiving supportive care, but not treatment, to prevent millions from becoming afflicted with the disease.'

The argument is false. There is a serious difficulty in using the 'triage' metaphor in AIDS policy. The reason (as Nicoli Nattrass points out) is that allocating resources between antiretroviral treatment and prevention is not a zero-sum game, in which the more you take from the one, the less the other gets. In fact, giving resources to both enhances each. Treatment and prevention are not competing, mutually cancelling strategies. They are complementary.

Fundamentally, those arguing against treatment suffered from a failure of belief in our capacity as humans to change the world in which we live. That world is very changeable. We can change it. The sceptical arguments ignored potential reductions in antiretroviral prices. Because activists campaigned, those price reductions in fact materialised. The sceptics even ignored technical arguments showing that mass treatment was feasible once the drop in antiretroviral prices was taken into account. They also failed to consider that a multilateral funding mechanism such as the Global Fund on AIDS, TB and Malaria could be created. Yet the fund now exists, and – however inadequately – it is addressing the practical problems of providing treatment in Africa and other resource-poor parts of the world.

The sceptics' lapses of imagination are not mere oversights. Activists campaigned for precisely these price reductions and for global funding. While the sceptics fretted about 'sustainability', activists made the changes happen. The truth is that the 'cost-effectiveness' argument suffered from its proponents' own lack of moral imagination.

A further truth is that the scepticism espoused sometimes seems to be compounded by the unexpressed reluctance some of its proponents feel in endorsing treatment options for those who have AIDS. The unspoken assumption is that their plight is their own fault, and that therefore they do not 'deserve' treatment.

In one of the United Kingdom's leading medical journals, a Cape Town philosopher, David Benatar, considered the contention that treatment is a basic and uniform human right. He argues that there is no moral obligation for government to treat those who contract HIV through 'negligence, indifference, arrogance or weakness'. Only because there are many people who contract HIV through no fault of their own, and because it is difficult or impossible for the public health system to differentiate between the 'responsible' and the 'irresponsible', should treatment be made universally available.

Among the 'innocent' Benatar includes children who receive the virus from their mothers, haemophiliacs, rape survivors, those who contracted the virus before the ways in which it is transmitted were known, as well as those who contract the disease even though they have taken reasonable precautions.

Included among the 'undeserving' are mothers of children with HIV, those who do not take precautions with multiple sex partners and 'those who force themselves on virgins in the erroneous and culpable belief that this will cure them of HIV'. Whether the mothers might themselves not have been 'innocently' infected is not explored. The writer agrees that there are good reasons for the state to provide social services for those who require them 'through no fault of their own'. By contrast, 'there is something ignominious about those who are responsible for their condition, and that of others, self-righteously joining the chorus of criticism [about government's failure to treat] if not leading the choir'.

The author's conception of 'innocence' and 'irresponsibility' betrays many problems. Even if we concede that the way in which many people acquire HIV may indeed be 'irresponsible', it is hard to see why this should justify denying them treatment that can save them from a terrible death. Does their 'irresponsibility' justly condemn them to the lingering suffering of death from AIDS?

Social services are a staple of the modern state. The admitted implication of the argument is that cigarette smokers, over-eaters, and self-injuring negligent drivers should be disbarred from healthcare. But we must take its implications further. What about those who become destitute because of their poor financial acumen or inability to do useful work? Should they, too, be denied social services? What about sportsmen, or even casual runners, who choose to exercise, and so develop injuries? And what about those who become sick because they do not exercise? Or those who over-exercise?

The modern welfare state extends protection to these people, even in the face of their own imprudence. The question is whether the fact that HIV is transmitted through 'irresponsible' acts that are sexual makes it easier for us to deny life-saving treatment to the poor. I think this is the case that is subtly being propounded. I think that sexual shame and rebuke still infests many of the arguments about 'irresponsibility' and 'sustainability'. This is external stigma re-surfacing again.

The real question is: how much humanity are we willing to muster in how we respond to stigma?

The argument is complicated by the fact that in the eyes of some the poor are ever undeserving. The argument about 'cost' is often an expedient that seeks to justify withholding available resources from poor people who are cast as 'undeserving' or 'irresponsible', or the authors of their own misfortune.

Paul Farmer explains how we use 'cost-effectiveness' as a rationale to cut back health benefits to the poor. Yet the poor are more likely to be sick than the non-poor. In this way, he says: 'We miss our chance to heal. In this setting, we're told, of 'scarce resources,' we imperil the health safety net. In the name of expedience, we miss our chance to be humane and compassionate.'

The one argument that seems least permissible and most insulting – and is easiest to refute – is that poor Africans are too unsophisticated to take the drugs they need to save their own lives.

The head of the United States Agency for International Development (USAID), Andrew Natsios, made some of the most unreflective – and rightly infamous – comments. In testimony before the US Congress in June 2001 he stated that treatment with antiretrovirals was impossible for Africans 'because of conflicts, because of lack of infrastructure, lack of doctors, lack of hospitals, lack of clinics, lack of electricity'. Africans, he claimed 'don't know what Western time is. You have to take these drugs a certain number of hours each day, or they don't work. Many people in Africa have never seen a clock or a watch their entire lives. And if you say, one o'clock in the afternoon, they do not know what you are talking about. They know morning, they know noon, they know evening, they know the darkness at night.'

These comments were silly. They were also demeaning – more demeaning to their author than to the poor people in Africa whose lives he presumed to talk about. But, tragically, they reportedly received support from a surprising and presumably unintended source: South African Health Minister Manto Tshabalala-Msimang. A well-known American health writer quoted her as stating (astutely) that complicated drug regimens cannot be taken in isolation. Instead, 'systems that . . . enable you to use the drugs' are essential. She was also reported to have said that 'if you have not started with infrastructure you will only make more problems'. So much was and is true. But Minister Tshabalala-Msimang regrettably added that many people needing AIDS drugs were in inaccessible villages – 'and many do not understand the importance of completing a course of drug therapy. People don't have watches.'

I reflected on the health minister's comments when I made the closing address at the Durban treatment conference in June 2002. Fearful of the government's seemingly deliberate tardiness in exploring antiretroviral options in dealing with the growing death toll from AIDS, these groupings brought together just under one thousand trade union members, health workers (including nurses, doctors and university professors), social workers, community organisers, activists and planners. Their self-imposed task was to put together a nationwide plan for implementing treatment through public health facilities.

That goal, I stated in closing, could readily be attained. Just eight years before, I pointed out, there had been no mobile phones in South Africa. Yet now there were more than ten million – many of them used by ordinary working and unemployed people in poor urban and rural areas. (The number of South African mobile phone users is now closer to fifteen million.) Cellphone technology was at the outset alien to all of us, I said, rich and poor, learned and unlearned. Yet we all now know, rich and poor, learned and unlearned, how to charge, encode and re-credit our phones, and how to message, send, receive, divert and forward calls.

It was, in short, silly to suggest that poor people, in Africa or elsewhere, could not apply learnable skills that they needed for the enhancement of their own lives.

No one suggests that sticking to an antiretroviral regimen is easy. Nor does anyone suggest that counselling, education and family and community support are not essential if AIDS treatments are to work in poor settings. Nontsikelelo herself confessed in her competition commission affidavit that in her first month on antiretroviral treatment she had had problems with adherence:

'I had a problem,' she said, 'of forgetting to take my pills during the first month, but I got used to them and committed myself to adhering since I knew that without them I would certainly die.'

Her story is now confirmed by the growing number of scientific studies of poor people on antiretroviral treatment. One important study at an antiretroviral programme in Somerset Hospital, Cape Town, found that poor people from the townships maintained excellent adherence to their medication programmes. The researchers pointed out that socio-economic position could not predict adherence. The most critical factor affecting adherence was the number of pills a patient had to take a day: the fewer tablets, the better the adherence.

Similarly successful treatment programmes have been implemented in all South Africa's major cities, as well as a small and poor rural district in the Eastern Cape province called Lusikisiki.

Elsewhere in Africa, a growing number of successful projects providing antiretroviral treatment to poor people, particularly in Botswana and Cameroon, disprove the sceptics' doubts about Africans' abilities to take their pills to save their own lives.

Brazil is often cited as a model of how a developing country can tackle the epidemic. Its per capita gross domestic product and socio-economic indicators are similar to South Africa's. There, over 100 000 people are on treatment. There is no reason why Brazil's success cannot be achieved throughout Africa. Indeed, in his state of the nation address in opening Parliament after the April 2004 elections, President Mbeki committed government to the aim of having more than 50 000 people on treatment through the public health sector by March 2005. Setting this target was vital, particularly since it was articulated by the president himself. And though it seems that the target will not be met, the reason will not be that poor people cannot take their medicines.

Stock shortages, poor counselling, the perpetuation of myths in communities – all these have bedevilled South Africa's recently started programme. But there is much encouraging news from health facilities that are implementing pilot programmes. If the will exists practical impediments to treatment can be overcome.

It is obviously true that many Africans – too many – live in desperately poor and often squalid living conditions. But it is patronising to presume that living in adversity disqualifies people from taking responsibility for their own lives by taking medicines properly. All medicating patients – rich and poor, African and non-African – need information, training, encouragement and support. They all deserve it, as well as the medications that make this backup necessary.

Throughout Africa, people needing antiretroviral treatment are demonstrating that they can save their own lives through daily action. It is a story as old as human life.

Of course it would be naïve simply to project success stories like that of Nontsikelelo Zwedala onto a whole community or a whole continent. Adherence to antiretroviral medication is not easy. The drugs must be taken regularly and timeously. Some of the drugs must be taken with, others without, or a specified number of hours before, or after, food – though such complexities have become rarer as the drugs themselves and the combinations have become simpler. But taking life-saving medication becomes particularly difficult where health systems are inadequate and living conditions hard. It is even more difficult when the disease is stigmatised, and when the patient lives in fear and isolation and silence.

But these conditions are contingent. They are subject to human change. We are capable of changing them. In Africa, the efforts of many health workers, government officials, community organisers and activists are changing them.

In addition to the fact that the drugs are difficult to take and that compliance with them may be difficult to secure, reactions to them may also be difficult to monitor. The treatment activists have never denied these difficulties. They have only insisted – rightly – that none of these problems render mass provision of treatment 'unsustainable'. But a further sombre reality is that the drugs are toxic. Their side effects can be dangerous. If not monitored and promptly dealt with, they can be fatal.

In April 2002, Sarah Hlalele died. Her death was particularly poignant. It sent shock waves through the community of people living with AIDS. Sarah had played a courageous part in the Treatment Action Campaign court case about preventing mother-to-child transmission of HIV. She made an affidavit describing herself a thirty-year-old woman resident in Sharpeville. 'At the moment,' she told the court, 'I do not have a permanent address. I was staying with my sister, but after I became sick my brother told people in the community that I have AIDS and now it is painful for me to live there. I am trying to find a shelter for my baby and myself.'

Although Sarah was a proud volunteer for and member of the TAC, she feared further victimization – and asked the court to treat her name as confidential and to refer to her only as 'SH'.

'I am the mother of two children. My first-born is a girl aged twelve. My son was born on 18 July 2001, and is presently in intensive care in Sebokeng hospital . . .When I became pregnant this year I first went to Natalspruit hospital in Thokoza . . . I knew about nevirapine for reducing the risk of my baby getting HIV from me. . . . I went to Chris Hani Baragwanath hospital (CHB) on 14 March 2001. At CHB they gave me a tablet of the drug called nevirapine. They wanted to give me some drops for the baby when it was born, but because they said the amount would depend on the weight of the baby I said I would come back after he was born. They said this must be before three days have passed. . . .

'On July 18th in the morning I had a severe pain, but I didn't think I was going to give birth as I was only seven months pregnant. I told my sister that I needed to go to the hospital and she called an ambulance . . . Because I did not know that I was in labour when the ambulance took me from home I did not bring the nevirapine tablet with me.

'At Sebokeng hospital I told the doctor that I was HIV positive. But they could not give me nevirapine because it was not available. I was very tired, as my recent illness had made me very weak.

'I gave birth to a boy. They took my baby away because he was very small. They told me he was in Ward 7. I still wanted my baby to have the nevirapine after he was born, but because he was so small they could not take him to CHB [where nevirapine was available]. I asked them for an ambulance, but found out that the hospital had arranged a bus to transport my premature baby to Chris Hani Baragwanath Hospital. I felt that this was not safe, so he did not receive the medicine.

'Now it is too late. It worries me to think that my baby didn't get the drops. I feel very angry. I don't want to think about whether my baby may be HIV positive. I have to wait for eighteen months until they can tell me. This is very painful.

'As a mother I believe that women, like me, who have HIV should have the right to take steps to try to protect our children.'

This brave account later helped secure a judgment on 5 July 2002 that compelled the South African government to make antiretroviral treatment available to women like Sarah. But a year after making her affidavit, Sarah herself was dead. At an anguished memorial service in an Anglican church in Yeoville, Johannesburg, I joined a speakers' roster of those recounting her agony, her courage, and her perseverance. Her doctor, Dr Francois Venter, also spoke. He explained that toxic reactions to the drugs can occur, particularly when patients' immune systems are severely weakened.

In Sarah's case, as her affidavit explained, she was being treated at Soweto's large public hospital, Chris Hani Baragwanath – a perilous two-hour journey from her home. It was hard for Sarah to travel, and the side effects the drugs were having on her were not promptly monitored and dealt with. In a radio interview, Mark Heywood, AIDS Law Project leader, claimed that the aspersions ANC leader Peter Mokaba had cast on antiretroviral drugs in early 2002 had upset Sarah terribly. As a result she was reluctant to believe that she was experiencing side effects and left it too late before she tried to seek help.

Peter Mokaba himself died, reportedly of AIDS, just two months after Sarah, in June 2002.

A year after Sarah's death, another Treatment Action Campaign activist died of side effects caused by antiretroviral treatment. She was Charlene Wilson, a lovely, gently spoken woman with braided hair from the Pretoria east mixed-race community of Eersterust. She started treatment in October 2002. Her CD4 count was below ten and she was already very ill. Initially, she improved. But within a few months she fell victim to lactic acidosis, a dangerous build-up of acids in the blood which sometimes comes as a side effect of stavudine [d4T] and didanosine.

By the time Charlene was diagnosed as having lactic acidosis, it was irreversible. She was admitted to the Helen Joseph Hospital's HIV clinic in Johannesburg's western suburbs, where Sister Sue Roberts, a pioneer in treating AIDS in the public health system, battled in vain to reverse the increasingly toxic reaction of her blood.

In his radio interview after Sarah Hlalele's death, Mark Heywood said that the problem of side effects should not inhibit treatment provision. 'We have known about side effects for as long as we have known about these drugs. Not all people suffer these side effects. The key things are patient and doctor education. I do think Sarah was a heroine and this is what she would have wanted us to learn from her death.'

That, too, was what Charlene Wilson's mother, Louisa Wilson, believed. She affirmed that when Charlene started on antiretroviral treatment she was close to death; late though it was, it gave Charlene six extra months of life.

Large-scale treatment access in the developing world and in South Africa in particular is still not an accomplished fact. Only about two per cent of the tens of millions of people in Africa living with AIDS are currently receiving antiretroviral treatment. Most of these are in South Africa.

Most South Africans currently on antiretroviral treatment pay privately for it or – like me – receive it with the help of their private healthcare insurance. South Africa's public programme still does not seem to have sufficient high-level backing. Activists and healthcare workers still have to cajole and push the national Department of Health.

Internationally, the GFATM remains critically underfunded. Despite the outspoken efforts of Richard Feachem, the head of the global fund, and of Stephen Lewis, the UN Secretary-General's special envoy on AIDS in Africa – who speaks passionately of the rich world's 'genocide by indifference' – the WHO goal of making treatment available to three million people by the end of 2005 seems only remotely possible.

It would be an over-simplification to argue that the lack of political will to make the necessary finance available is the only reason for these shortcomings. But it is the primary reason. For, to paraphrase John Kenneth Galbraith, when it comes to making money available to needy people, nothing is so firmly accepted by the well off 'as the damaging effect of money on the poor. We are at our most righteously compassionate in our concern for what unearned income will do to the unfortunate.'

As for the 'sustainability' of antiretroviral treatment programmes in poor countries, the best answer is provided by Paul Farmer, who has a gift not only for principled action but pithy expression:

'What, then, is not sustainable? It is not the cost of HIV treatment that is not sustainable; it's rather the opposition to treatment in high-burden areas that is not sustainable. It's not morally sustainable, it's not intellectually sustainable, it's not epidemiologically or socially sustainable.'

8 | Choices

On my sister Jeanie's eleventh birthday, when I was seven, my sister Laura was killed in a cycling accident. It was during our first family visit to Pretoria after our long first year in the children's home. It happened only days before the three of us were due to return by train to the institution. Laura was twelve. She was baking cookies for Jeanie's special day. The ingredients at my aunt Lydia's home, where we were staying, lacked only golden syrup. With a few coins from my mother's younger sister, Laura picked up a cousin's bicycle and set out for the nearby shop. At the stop street around the corner she met her death, killed instantly when a passing delivery van felled her.

There was no prosecution. She must have gone through the stop.

Of the dead speak no ill: but in Laura's case the injunction was superfluous. She was popular, conscientious, clever, industrious and, in our fractured family circumstances, parental to Jeanie and to me. For my mother, she ran errands and did the shopping, calming her when drink degraded my father to dissipation and destruction. When Jeanie and I squabbled she restored peace, wisely and fairly.

The bleak incomprehensible first year in Queenstown, hundreds of kilometres from family, where we were separated into three hostels, she with the older and Jeanie with the younger girls, and I with the younger boys, was eased by her fostering love and practical good sense. We would meet after school on the gravel hockey field beyond the hostels, or on the lawn next to the fields where the handyman-gardener Wilson – he was only ever 'Wilson' – cultivated vegetables. She excelled in her last year at the local school: a model student, all the teachers said, outstanding academically and showing high promise in leadership.

Now she was dead. It was impossible to understand the obliteration of her life. I remember the life-shifting moment when the neighbour's son ran into the yard where Jeanie and I were playing with our cousins and their friends, heavy with the horror and excitement of his news: something had happened to the girl staying with the family; there had been an accident on the corner; the 'tannie' (auntie) had to come quickly. Quickly.

My mother left in panic with my aunt. We were told to stay. Long hours later she returned, sedated and dazed. Laura was dead. She had accompanied her in the ambulance to the hospital, but it was already too late. Jeanie and I sought comfort behind my mother's back in a darkened bedroom, the living room hushed with the shocked murmuring of visitors and family.

At the funeral my father sat in the back row, a desolate figure between two men in uniform. He was spending the year in Sonderwater Prison in Cullinan outside Pretoria. We were not told why. The prison commander gave him special dispensation to wear civilian clothes for the funeral. But he was not allowed to join the procession to the grave in Pretoria West's Zandfontein cemetery. Later, my mother told us he was serving a sentence for car theft.

Sonderwater means 'Waterless'. But my father spent the year productively, carpentering little wooden gifts. Two decades before, while still a teenager, he had joined the volunteer South African army sent north to fight Nazism. Severely wounded in his left leg, and held for years as a prisoner of war in North Africa and Italy, he returned, his family told us, changed: one of the changes was a severe alcohol dependency from which it seemed he could find no escape. After his release from prison he resumed his life cycle: earning good wages as an electrician, then after a few months losing his job when he went on a sodden binge, from which only the nadir of utter destitution ever seemed to bring reprieve.

A few days after the funeral we returned to the home. The Eastern Cape schools were starting the new term. My mother obtained money for a train ticket to accompany Jeanie and me on the grinding overnight journey. The staff and the other children received us kindly, even respectfully – we were the Camerons, whom something incomprehensibly important had befallen: our sister had just been killed. It was as if it had happened to someone else.

Seeing their responses, I sensed that events had two layers: the inner and the outer. I could deal with the outer. I was the boy whose elder sister had been tragically killed. Immersing myself in my books, I turned to excelling at school. Intellectual achievement pointed away from the unbearable.

Jeanie nearly failed her next school year. Though she too blocked off too many feelings, she grieved deeply for Laura. Moving closer to me, her love shielded me protectively in the next years. We are photographed in our first winter together in Queenstown after Laura's death, my right shoulder scrunched against her pre-pubescent chest, her left hand – her good hand, her primary hand, for using which she was beaten in her early years at school – pulling my left shoulder protectively toward her. The hand has remained.

In the wake of Laura's death and the final break-up of our family that preceded it, I took recourse to a childish world of fantasy. Except when actually reading or studying, or when the company of other people forced me to engage, I was absorbed by a vibrant world of my own creation, one peopled with figures and events and achievements that numbed all shock and pain. The fantasies kept their grip on me for decades into adulthood. They were to be my psychic location for much of the next thirty years. I did not grieve for Laura. I did not have to. It had happened to someone else.

Years later, a wise and patient professional counsellor named Anthony Hamburger coaxed me gently from that world into the risks and pain and vexation and occasional joy of ordinary living. One night at home during this arduous process, more than three decades after Jeanie's eleventh birthday, I pictured Laura's death for the first time. The access of horror I had been unable to feel as a child now brought me to the floor. For the first time grief wracked my body. Grief, and – startlingly – a choking rage: why had Laura not been more careful? Why had she not stopped at the sign, checked the traffic, avoided the van? How could she leave us when we needed her so?

For years Jeanie and I kept our time in the home a secret. We felt ashamed, soiled, disadvantaged. When the director of the Johannesburg Guild Cottage children's home and treatment centre for abused children, Zelda Kruger, asked me to talk at their annual donors' and volunteers' function in 1996, I accepted. In speaking about children's rights under our constitution – the indicated topic – I underscored their importance by relating them to some of my own experiences at the children's home. I did so understatedly and, in keeping with the occasion, professionally: safely. But for me their mere mention was a breakthrough.

Later, a group of our contemporaries in the home started an email list. They tracked me down and listed me before they got to Jeanie, who had assumed her married name. At first she couldn't bear to open the messages I forwarded to her. Later she wrote to thank the organisers: 'For me personally it has been a great help in coming to terms with the past. Despite my "unhappy childhood" I've managed to make a success of my life . . . I have everything I could possibly want in life: a loving family, good health, fitness, money, an interesting job, education, leisure, a home, lots of travel and holidays . . .' Yet amidst this plenty she realised that she needed help in dealing with our past: 'Psychologists say that unfinished business (trauma or grief you haven't worked through) is a major cause of depression in later years. I seem to have coped with unhappiness in my childhood by blocking off the memories of my father's abandonment, my sister's death, and the home. It's something I never used to talk about. I felt so inferior that I didn't want people to be prejudiced by knowing I came from a children's home.'

'When I at last started reading the emails, a wonderfully healing process began. The names I recognise are bringing back good memories. I realise the home was not something to be ashamed of.' For Jeanie, posting her email was a breakthrough. Her speaking out emboldened others to do so too, and she strongly encouraged the suggestion that we should hold a reunion at the home.

In September 2004, thirty of us, children from the 1960s, re-united in Queenstown. Now adults, we were connected only by memory and experience to the buildings that now serve as hostels for the local boys' school. Asked to speak on behalf of all, I made my theme choices: choices that lead to integration or disintegration. Forty years ago we had found ourselves in Queenstown involuntarily, placed in the home because of choices that our parents and other people had made: often bad choices, choices that too often were destructive and damaging and disintegrating for us. Those choices had in many cases injured our lives. And our memories of that time often represented pain and difficulty. And yet we had survived. Not only survived, but survived to be able to make more constructive choices for our own lives.

Our reunion brought us together, I said, because of the positive choices that we had been able to make for ourselves. Our decision to be with each other represented an integrating and life-enhancing choice for each of us. It meant that we recognised and respected the importance to our lives of our time in the home, and the importance of our friendship and bonds with those who were with us there so many decades ago. And so, I said, we derived strength and wholeness from each other, and from the love and truth that our gathering represented in each of our lives.

For the adult children from the home, pain, grief, the stigma of poverty and destitution, an amputating bereavement, have been turned by healing action into part of the complex, often sad, sometimes joyful, ordinary struggle that is our daily living.

Against Africa's arduous and sometimes bloody struggle for its humanity over the last half-century, against its people's poverty and bereavements, the personal adversities of a group of destitute white children at a rural institution in the 1960s do not rate high in the order of calamity. Those now on the mailing list seem to have jobs, homes with running water and generated power, access to electronic communication. Apartheid's privileges have played their part, as they have in my life.

My burning belief that actions can change social patterns and the lives they determine, that government and human institutions are duty bound to address disadvantage and redress injustice where they occur, was seared into me by the benefits just such interventions accorded my own life. Four rich years at one of the country's best whites-only boys' high schools, followed by a privileged university education – also whites-only – opened a world of opportunity to me that during the years in the home I could not have dreamed would ever be accessible. I see all too vividly how other young lives, trapped in similar adversity or far worse, would flourish were Africa's social institutions to provide for them the opportunities that life opened to me.

AIDS is only one of Africa's current adversities. There are also wars and bloodshed and famine and oppression. And Africa's adversities are only part of a perilous world in which excess of power (too often driven by religious extremism: Christian, Muslim and Jewish) creates injustices that quell human flourishing.

But amidst all these others AIDS is an important adversity, important morally and practically and socially, because it tells us so much about ourselves and about our other problems. Our responses to a sexually transmitted disease that is potentially fatal show us how much the facts of sex and death still provoke fear and flight, rather than understanding and acceptance, in our cultures. Our responses to a disease whose greatest impact is now on poor black Africans tell us much about our attitudes to poverty and to race.

AIDS over the last twenty-five years has cast a sharp light on medical practice, scientific discovery, government power and extragovernmental activism. It has led to an irreversible shift in the relationship between medical science and the public, changing the way in which consumers and wielders of medical and scientific knowledge see each other and deal with each other. The consumers have made significant gains, from which all have benefited. In Western societies, patients have more power, more knowledge, more assertive courage, more dignity, than before the epidemic.

AIDS has also raised fundamental questions about corporate profits and the exploitation of knowledge in the public good: those who claim to use exclusive legal license for the public benefit must demonstrate that they are truly acting in its interests. If not, they deserve our wrath, and their privilege of exclusivity should be revoked or its extent curbed.

In Africa, too, AIDS has changed the way we see the responsibilities of corporations in reacting to poverty and illness. The struggle to end denial of AIDS treatments to Africa's millions was necessary because the initial position of corporate leaders and shareholders in the West, backed by their governments, was simple: they were entitled to ex-act maximum profits on their medications in Western market con-ditions. Yet those conditions systematically excluded Africa from fair access to the very same markets, while systematically depriving it of fair compensation for its raw materials and labour. Africa's pover-ty is no doubt in part attributable to the greed and short-sightedness and folly and hubris of some of its leaders. But in much larger meas-ure it is an outcome of a history that the West has imposed on Africa, and a present the West continues to impose on it, through a world economic order that deprives its peoples of opportunity to partici-pate with dignity on terms of just equality.

We live in a contorted world, where some – including myself – live in relative affluence and comfort, our health secured by medical at-tention and access to care and treatments. Others live in grotesquely contrasting poverty, deprived of the essentials of life. Is this a 'nat-ural' order of things? Before the AIDS epidemic it was easier to think so. Those living in affluence often do not see, still less have any con-tact with, people suffering from preventable illness, avoidable hunger and remediable destitution. Or they think of them as less deserv-ing, or of their condition as self-inflicted. Certainly they acknowl-edge no functional connection between the prosperity of the West and the impoverishment of the rest. Distance, ideology and the in-evitable frailties of human understanding and connection help main-tain comfort.

But AIDS has helped pierce the insulation. The epidemic's prox-imities and juxtapositions have brought the inequalities of the de-veloped and developing world closer than comfort can warrant.

In the affluent northern hemisphere of the 1980s, the public wit-nessed tens and hundreds of thousands of gay men suffering and dying, gay men who fought with passion to re-order human struc-tures and attitudes and policies that denied them dignity and treat-ment. Their struggle was unexpectedly, abundantly rewarded. Treat-ment arrived: and the wealth of the developed world reduced their death and suffering to a fraction of what had gone before.

Now in the 1990s and the early 2000s, the world witnesses poor black people in Africa dying of the same condition. The same viral particles. The same physiological effects. The same symptoms. The same suffering. The same ghastly, lingering fleshly surcease. Only different countries, different colours, different people. For too many it had to begin to seem intolerable. And unnecessary. The drama and horror of the epidemic began to bridge the imaginative distance between the way 'we' can live and the way others must live.

The claim of 'entitlement' underlying drug pricing and availability encompassed a protective moral comfort, a defensive ethical shielding, that had to be stripped off the positions and individuals they sheltered. Those claims endorsed as axiomatic propositions about the replication and use of human knowledge that in their application to Africa's epidemic were demonstrably outrageous. But the demonstration had to be made, gruellingly, and the change was (and sometimes still is) fiercely resisted. The exponents of the self-entitling propositions had to be exposed to public view, and their defences had to be subjected to public censure, the laws and policies and practices they supported humanely altered.

The rank immorality of the notion that tens of millions of poor people should be denied access to available medications because of limitations on the use of human knowledge had to be pronounced: and the opposition to the immorality had to prevail. And the successful assertion of the counter-view had to be carried through into practical effect. That last was and remains the most important task.

That process is still occurring. On its successful completion – on the practical implementation of what one writer has called 'the most extensive humanitarian venture in human history' – depends many millions of lives.

AIDS has cast unremitting light also on the influence and power that governments and leaders wield in Africa. Some leaders – in countries like Uganda, Botswana, Kenya – have responded to the grief and devastation of the epidemic with the resolution to include it in their plans for daily life. They have sought to 'normalise' the epidemic. They have done so by speaking about it, by getting others to speak about it, by including it as an elementary and ever-present and rightly obtrusive part of their policies and proposals and practices.

Others, including those in my own country, have struggled to accept that a virally borne, mostly sexually transmitted, epidemic of suffering and death confronts us. They have sought to blank out an anguish that is too hideous to bear, yet has proved too encompassing to ignore.

In South Africa, a challenge to the medical science of AIDS that sought to defend the humanity and dignity of Africans led instead to a tragic delay in concerted action during which many African lives have been lost amidst hideous individual suffering. A resistance to conventional thinking that was meant to defy crass stereotypes about African sexuality led to a moralising re-emphasis on sex and sexuality that in practice served to inhibit behaviour change – just as workers were struggling to help those at risk to deal rationally and autonomously with the sexual and social roles and responsibilities and vulnerabilities that spur the epidemic. Stigma and denial were unexpectedly enhanced. The consequences have been devastating.

AIDS has pitched our continent into a vast agony of mourning. Every family, every workplace, every sphere of every human organisation in central and southern Africa has felt the epidemic's seeping of strength, its obtrusion of ghastly and disfiguring symptoms, its premature bereavements, its copious and often untended product of parentless young. And many of us, too many, have reacted mutely. We have responded to the epidemic with silence; and our doing so has rendered it and those who suffer under it unspeakable. We have too often placed those suffering the effects of the virus beyond the reach of our embrace, beyond word and comfort and help and remedy.

But we will not be whole as a continent until we have lived and fully held and endured and dealt with the total largeness of the calamity that the disease has brought upon us. Our country will not be whole until we have sought to understand and have confronted and dealt with our own fears and failures and denials in dealing with the epidemic.

I know that I have AIDS. I know it every day, every hour, in my working and thinking and playing. I feel it as I take my tablets twice daily,

213

as I wait with repressed but still perceptible anxiety for my doctor's call after my twice-yearly blood checks, when I watch heart in mouth for news of fresh breakthroughs in viral knowledge and treatment that may hold benefit for me and others. I know it too when I see increasing numbers of gaunt, energyless fellow South Africans who lack the access and benefits and protections I enjoy. I know it when I hear of friends and acquaintances who, too fearful to be diagnosed and treated, withdraw wastingly, wastefully, from help and health, because we have not invested them with enough belief in their own power to live and to be loved.

I carry in me now, a memory like blood, the shock of my own diagnosis, the long years of muteness and secrecy, the fear of fleshly failure, the allies I harboured and nurtured within of the stigmas and hatreds outside. I know that I have AIDS. It is not just that I refuse to forget. It's that I cannot. Remembering is in me, like blood.

And yet my days also have sun and food and energy and fun and work and friendship and family and hope and challenge and belief and happiness. I feel joy to be gainfully occupied within a large, ambitious and improbable project – a journey of transformation that beckons South Africans beyond the demeaning structures within which our history sought to confine us. I feel joy to have life in a country and a continent where human life started, where human life continues, and where human life can flourish more fully if we believe enough in our own capacity to achieve it.

We cannot escape our grief or the losses we have experienced or the suffering that has been. But we can act to minimise those occurring now, to prevent further deaths, to open our hearts and hold in them those who, now, are afflicted with illness and its isolation. Our grief is there. It is continent-wide, pandemic. But we cannot allow our grief and our bereavement to inflict a further loss upon us: the loss of our own full humanity, our capacity to feel and respond and support. We must incorporate our grief into our everyday living, by turning it into energy for living, by exerting ourselves as never before.

AIDS is above all a remediable adversity. Our living and our life forces are stronger, our capacity for wholeness as humans is larger, than the individual effects of the virus. Africa seeks healing. That healing lies within the power of our own actions. In inviting us to deal with the losses it has already inflicted, and, more importantly, in enjoining us to avoid future losses that our own capacity to action make unnecessary, AIDS beckons us to the fullness and power of our own humanity. It is not an invitation that we should avoid or refuse.

Notes

EPIGRAPH

Primo Levi, Afterword to *If This is a Man* and *The Truce* (Abacus edition, 2003), p. 390.

CHAPTER ONE

1. The motorcar fraud case is *Wayne Scholtz v The State*, appeal A453/97, October 1997, Witwatersrand Local Division of the High Court. My senior colleague was Mr Justice Dirk Marais. The three judges who decided the re-hearing in favour of the appellant accused were Judge-President Eloff, Mr Justice Goldblatt and Ms Justice Snyders.
2. According to the South African Institute of Race Relations, www.sairr.org.za, the per capita gross domestic product for South Africa in 1997 was R14 291. The gross national product was R13 422. Average monthly earnings per employee in the formal non-agricultural business sector were R3 890. I am grateful to the director, Mr John Kane-Berman, for extracting these figures for me.
3. Information on PCP from the website of the Centers for Disease Control, http://www.dpd.cdc.gov/dpdx/html/Pneumocystis.htm, accessed on 22 September 2003.
4. For information on the ANC's and the PAC's differing approaches to the liberation struggle in South Africa, see Tom Lodge, *Black Politics in South Africa Since 1945* (Ravan Press, 1983) p. 241ff.
5. The injustice of the South African courts' treatment of the Sharpeville Six is considered at greater length (together with other judicial failures) in the Bentham lecture, delivered at University College, London, on 23 March 2004, and published in (2004) 111 *South African Law Journal* 580; http://www.ucl.ac.uk/bentham.
6. The minister's and the judges' attacks on me for my participation in the campaign to save the Sharpeville Six, and my other criticisms of apartheid judges, are documented and considered in an article by the late Professor Etienne Mureinik, 'Law and Morality in South Africa' (1988) 105, *South African Law Journal* 457. This article formed the basis for Professor Mureinik's speech at the colloquium mentioned in the text.
7. My academic article criticising the verdict is in (1988) *South African Journal for Criminal Justice* 258.
8. Prakash Diar wrote a moving testimony: *The Sharpeville Six* (McLelland & Stewart, London and Toronto, 1990).
9. The bitter counterattack by the appeal court judge who wrote the verdict in the Sharpeville Six case is in *S v Mgedezi and others* (1989) (1) South African Law Reports 687 (A) on p. 702. I riposted in (1989) *Annual Survey of South African Law* 598.

10. The Six were released from prison in 1991 as part of a deal between the outgoing apartheid government and the African National Congress. Their personal testimonies at meetings and on television programmes have kept the case in the popular mind.

11. For an illuminating account of how public interest lawyers used the apartheid legal system in the 1980s to advance liberation goals, see Richard L Abel: *Politics by Other Means – Law in the Struggle against Apartheid 1980-1994* (Routledge, New York and London, 1995).

12. The statute that prohibited all workplace testing for HIV without the consent of the Labour Court is the Employment Equity Act 55 of 1998. Section 6(1) expressly prohibits 'unfair discrimination' on the ground of 'HIV status', while section 7(2) prohibits testing of an employee to establish that employee's HIV status unless the Labour Court deems it justifiable. Job applicants are included in the definition of 'employee'.

CHAPTER TWO

1. Websites with facts on AIDS include http://www.aidsmap.com/, http://www.aegis.org/, http://www.cdc.gov/hiv/dhap.htm, http://www.avert.org/, http://www.thebody.com/index.shtml.

2. Recent research on improvements in morbidity and mortality as a result of antiretroviral drug regimens reflected in A Mocroft and others 'Decline in the AIDS and death rates in the EuroSIDA study: an observational study', *The Lancet* vol. 362 Issue 9377 p.22.

3. Information on bubonic plague from http://www.cdc.gov/ncidod/dvbid/plague/.

4. Meanings of 'shame' and 'stigma' adapted from the Shorter Oxford English Dictionary.

5. Information on Botswana government's 'opt-out' approach to HIV testing, applied since January 2004, available from http://www.health-e.org.za/news/article_audio.php?uid=20031143.

6. On apartheid law and resistance to it through law, a reference to Richard L Abel: *Politics by Other Means – Law in the Struggle against Apartheid 1980-1994* (Routledge, New York and London, 1995) is again appropriate.

7. The shameful history of the repatriation of nearly 1 000 Malawian mineworkers in 1987/1988 is fully documented in E Cameron & E Swanson 'Restrictions on Migrant Workers, Immigrants and Travellers with HIV or AIDS: South Africa's Step Forward' (1992) 13, South African *Industrial Law Journal* 496-500.

8. A helpful discussion of stigma is by Jeanine Cogan and Gregory Herek in the *Encyclopedia of AIDS*, http://www.thebody.com/encyclo/stigma.html, accessed 15 October 2003. Prof Herek has written widely on the subject: http://psychology.ucdavis.edu/herek.

9. The book of essays on gay and lesbian lives in South Africa is by Mark Gevisser and Edwin Cameron: *Defiant Desire – Gay and Lesbian Lives in South Africa* (published in South Africa by Ravan Press, 1994 and in the United States by Routledge, 29 West 35th St, New York, NY 10001).

10. *Hoffmann v South African Airways* is reported in 2001 (1) SA 1 (CC); 2000 (11) BCLR 1235 (CC) and can be accessed at http://www.concourt.gov.za/judgment.php?case_id=12079.

11. Mr Graham McIntosh, MP, of the opposition Democratic Party, wrote to the *Natal Mercury* on 30 April 1999, stating that 'Judge Edwin Cameron's HIV/AIDS infection is a logical consequence of his self-proclaimed, public and enthusiastic support for and practice of a homosexual orientation'. A media statement dated 10 May 1999 by Mr Douglas Gibson MP, Democratic Party Federal Council Chairperson, recorded Mr McIntosh's public apology.

12. Information on Botswana from UNAIDS, Irin News http://www.irinnews.org/AIDSreport.asp?ReportID = 2089&SelectRegion = Southern Africa&SelectCountry = BOTSWANA, accessed on 15 October 2003, and Geoff Dyer '2 in 5' *Financial Times Magazine* October 11, 2003, issue no 25.

13. According to the IFPMA (International Federation of Pharmaceutical Manufacturers Associations) as of March 2004 more than 15 000 Botswanans (Batswana) were receiving medication and 25 000 were actually enrolled in the MASA program. At that time they expected 1 000 new patients to be enrolled each month in the programme. See www.ifpma.org/Health/hiv/health_achap_hiv.aspx, accessed on 5 August 2004.

14. Information on Zambia from UNAIDS and the Zambian AIDS Law Research and Advocacy Network at http://www.zaran.org.

15. The address by Chief Justice Sakala on Saturday 21 June 2003 is available at http://www.zaran.org/judgesreport.html.

16. Gladwell told me that he came from a Zulu-speaking part of northeast South Africa. My scepticism was aroused when the police repeatedly arrested him as an illegal immigrant. But arrest on trumped-up charges of immigrancy befalls many black South Africans. So when Gladwell produced what seemed to be an authentic identity document, I referred him to a colleague at the Wits law clinic. Sued for wrongful arrest, the police gave Gladwell a favourable settlement of several thousands.

CHAPTER THREE

1. *Titus Andronicus* at the Royal Shakespeare Theatre, Stratford on Avon, from 12 December 2003, directed by Bill Alexander. Joe Dixon played Aron.

2. Mozart's *Magic Flute* at Covent Garden, June 2003.

3. Material on the British response to AIDS, and High Commissioner Kelvin White's 1986 despatch on AIDS from Lusaka, from Virginia Berridge: *AIDS in the UK – The Making of Policy, 1981-1994* (Oxford University Press, 1996).

4. Material on the early United States response to AIDS from Randy Shilts: *And the Band Played On* (Penguin, 1987), p. 586: 'No hint that the disease might spread to straights, no matter how specious, was too small to put on page one.'

5. AIDS as the product of gay lifestyle choices and 'the long-term consumption of recreational drugs': Peter Duesberg and David Rasnick, 'The AIDS dilemma: Drug diseases blamed on a passenger virus' (1998) 104 (2) *Genetica* 85.

6. Figures on international prevalence of HIV taken from UNAIDS, AIDS epidemic update, December 2002, available at http://www.UNAIDS.org/html/pub/Publications/IRC-pub03/epiupdate2002, and from *Report on the Global HIV/AIDS Epidemic 2002* (UNAIDS/02/26E, English original July 2002).

7. Material on India from the Country AIDS Policy Analysis Project of the University of California San Francisco's AIDS Research Institute (AIDS Policy Research Center) Report 'HIV/AIDS in India', August 2003, available at http://ari.ucsf.edu/ARI/policy/profiles/India.

8. In a special lead article on AIDS in India in its 17 April 2004 issue, *The Economist* continued to warn against insufficient government action and commitment: 'Against such a background, forecasts of millions more infections seem horribly plausible. Yet similar forecasts were made for Thailand and Brazil – and were proved wrong, thanks to committed intervention.'

9. On Friday 9 January 2004 the BBC reported the Kenyan household survey that suggest-

ed that the UNAIDS prevalence estimates might be overstated. See http://news.bbc.co.uk/go/em/fr/-/2/hi/health/3379707.stm, accessed on 9 January 2004.

10. Information on Cameroon health ministry's 2003/2004 national survey from United Nations PlusNews (Office for the Coordination of Humanitarian Affairs Integrated Regional Information Network), 29 October 2004.

11. Rian Malan, 'Africa isn't dying of AIDS', *The Spectator*, 14 December 2003, accessed at http://www.spectator.co.uk/article.php3?table=old&section=current&issue=2003-12-13&id=3830 on 15 December 2003, preceded by Rian Malan 'AIDS in Africa – In search of the truth', *Rolling Stone Magazine*, 22 November 2001, available on the denialist website: www.virusmyth.net/aids/data/rmafrica.htm [accessed 4 June 2003].

12. Nathan Geffen, National Manager of Treatment Action Campaign, 'Rian Malan Spreads Confusion about AIDS Statistics', posted to www.tac.org.za on 23 January 2004.

13. Randy Shilts, *And the Band Played On*, p. 19: '. . . sex was part and parcel of political liberation'.

14. Information on Saartjie Baartman from President Thabo Mbeki's 'Letter from the President', 10 May 2002, www.anc.org.za/ancdocs/anctoday/2002/at19.htm#, and published in *ANC TODAY*, Volume 2, No. 19, May 10-16, 2002; and is also available at http://web.mit.edu/racescience/in_media/baartman/baartman_mbekiletter.htm.

15. Anonymous, 'Castro Hlongwane, Caravans, Cats, Geese, Foot & Mouth and Statistics – HIV/AIDS and the Struggle for the Humanisation of the African', (March 2002). Authorship of this document was claimed by prominent ANC activist Mr Peter Mokaba, MP, who died shortly after (reportedly of AIDS-related causes), but this has been doubted: see Howard Barrell 'Would the real Aids dissident please declare himself?' *Mail & Guardian*, 19 April 2002, and Jaspreet Kindra, 'A refreshing willingness to engage,' *Mail & Guardian*, 14 June 2002.

16. President Mbeki on representations of Africans as 'germ carriers, and human beings of a lower order that cannot subject its passions to reason': Inaugural ZK Mathews Memorial Lecture, University of Fort Hare, 12 October 2001, http://www.anc.org.za/ancdocs/history/mbeki/2001/tm1012.html [11 June 2004].

17. Information on the fourteenth century plague from Philip Ziegler, *The Black Death* (Collins, 1969), p. 115: 'The Atlantic coast of Spain was less severely affected than the Mediterranean. Portugal as a whole did not suffer particularly seriously'. P. 116: 'Certain areas escaped lightly. Bohemia, large areas of Poland, a mysterious pocket between France, Germany and the Low Countries, tracts of the Pyrenees. . . . Even today, the science of epidemiology can't provide a full conclusive answer.'

CHAPTER FOUR

1. President Thabo Mbeki: 'there . . . exists a large volume of scientific literature alleging that, among other things, the toxicity of this drug [AZT] is such that it is in fact a danger to health.' Hansard, National Council of Provinces, Thursday 28 October 1999; see www.anc.org.za/ancdocs/history/mbeki/1999/tm1028.html [17 June 2003].

2. Evidence establishing the causal link between HIV and AIDS is collected in National Institutes of Health / National Institute of Allergy and Infectious Diseases Fact Sheet, *The Evidence that HIV Causes AIDS*, available at www.niaid.nih.gov/factsheets/evidhiv.htm [4 June 2003]. A good sampling of denialist views can be obtained on the website www.virusmyth.com.

3. The 'hypothesis' of HIV as the cause of AIDS, and AIDS deaths in Africa, as 'a minor fraction of conventional mortality under a new name'; 'non-contagious risk factors that are limited to certain sub-sets of the African population'; 'deceptive AIDS propaganda' alleging the existence of a microbial AIDS epidemic in Africa has been 'introduced and inspired by new American biotechnology', one that – at least in the case of HIV testing – 'provides job security' for virologists and doctors, 'without ever producing any public health benefits': Peter Duesberg and David Rasnick, 'The AIDS dilemma: drug diseases blamed on a passenger virus' (1998) 104 (2) *Genetica* 85, and Peter Duesberg, *The African AIDS epidemic: New and contagious - or - old under a new name?* (Submission to President Mbeki's AIDS Panel, 22 June 2000) available at www.duesberg.com/subject/africa2.html [4 June 2003].
4. Presidential spokesman Parks Mankahlana quoted as describing the remit of the presidential AIDS panel as 'whether there is this thing called AIDS, what it is, whether HIV leads to AIDS, whether there is something called HIV', in Mark Schoofs, 'Flirting with Pseudoscience', *Village Voice*, 21 March 2000.
5. President Mbeki's letter to Western leaders was quoted extensively in the *Washington Post* of Wednesday 19 April 2000.
6. Cabinet statements on HIV/AIDS of 17 April 2002 available at www.gov.za/speeches/cabinetaids02.htm [17 June 2003]; and of 9 October 2002 available at www.gov.za/issues/hiv/cabinetaids9oct02.htm [17 June 2003]. The latter indicates that 'Government is actively engaged in addressing these challenges, in order to create the conditions that would make it feasible and effective to use antiretrovirals in the public health sector'.
7. The 'wild and insulting claims about the African and Haitian origins of HIV': letter by President Mbeki to leader of the official opposition Tony Leon, carried in the Johannesburg *Sunday Times* 9 July 2000.
8. Professor William Makgoba's editorial was in *Science* magazine, 2000, May 19; 288:1171 – accessed at http://www.sciencemag.org, on 23 September 2003.
9. Archbishop Njongonkulu Ndungane: 'SA's AIDS policy is sinful, says Archbishop', Johannesburg *Star*, 25 January 2002, http://www.iol.co.za/index.php?set_id+1&click_id=13&art_id=qw1011981601754B232.
10. Justice Malala, 'Down with the People', 'Insight' column in Johannesburg *Sunday Times*, 7 November 1999, http://www.suntimes.co.za/1999/11/07/insight/in06.htm; 'Mbeki's out fiddling a discordant tune while at home the AIDS crisis slowly burns', 'Clause 16' column, Johannesburg *Sunday Times*, 23 July 2000, http://www.suntimes.co.za/2000/07/23/insight/in03.htm; 'Another Country', *The Guardian*, Wednesday 14 April 2004, http://www.guardian.co.uk/aids/story/0,7369,1191298,00.htm.
11. Mondli Makhanya: 'Mister President, Your Country Needs You', Johannesburg *Sunday Times*, 24 September 2000.
12. Jovial Rantao: 'Talk, talk, talk. It's time to act on AIDS', Johannesburg *Star*, 25 July 2003, http://www.gate.cosatu.org.za/pipermail/news/2003-July/000268.html.
13. Khathu Mamaila: 'Pulling back the power curtain', Johannesburg *Star*, 9 December 2002, http://www.thestar.co.za/index.php?fSectionId=225&fArticleId=25091; 'AIDS studies should not stereotype', Johannesburg *Star*, 2 February 2004, http://www.thestart.co.za/index.php?fSectionId=225&fArticleId=338799.
14. Dr Kgositsile Letlape: 'Newsmaker', Johannesburg *Sunday Times* Business Times Section, 15 February 2004, profile by Chris Barron.
15. *The Durban Declaration: A Declaration by Scientists and Physicians affirming HIV is the*

Cause of AIDS (July 2000), reprinted in (2000) XIII (10) *Body Positive*, with a commentary by Raymond A Smith.

16. President Mbeki's address at the opening session of the XIII International Conference on AIDS, Durban, 9 July 2000 available at *www.anc.org.za/ancdocs/history/mbeki/2000/ tm0709.html* [5 June 2003].

17. Nkosi Johnson's work on AIDS, including his speech at the opening ceremony of the XIII International Conference on AIDS: See Jane Fox: *Nkosi's Story* (Spearhead, 2003).

18. 'The Deafening Silence of AIDS' [First Jonathan Mann Memorial Lecture at the XIII International Conference on AIDS and HIV, Durban, July 2000], *Health and Human Rights* vol. 5 no. 1 Autumn 2000 (Harvard University) pp. 7-24.

19. The Constitutional Court judgment outlawing discrimination by South African Airways (a state agency) against a work-seeker with HIV: *Hoffmann* v *South African Airways* 2001 (1) SA Law Reports 1 (CC), delivered 28 September 2000 per Ngcobo, J, on behalf of a unanimous Court, available at http://www.concourt.gov.za/judgment.php?case_id=12079.

20. The MTCT (nevirapine) case: *Minister of Health and others v Treatment Action Campaign and others* 2002 (5) SA Law Reports 721 (CC), available at http://www.concourt.gov.za/ judgment.php?case_id=11915.

21. Health minister Tshabalala-Msimang's attack on nevirapine and the Constitutional Court order at Bangkok international AIDS conference, July 2004: 'Tshabalala-Msimang renews attack on anti-AIDS drug', Johannesburg *Business Day*, 12 July 2004, http://www.bday.co.za/ bday/content/direct/1,3523,1656800-6078-0,00.html.

22. AIDS as a disease of 'of poverty and underdevelopment': President Mbeki 'Response to the Parliamentary Debate on the State of the Nation Address', National Assembly, 18 February 2003, available at www.anc.org.za/ancdocs/history/mbeki/2003/tm0218.html [5 June 2003]: 'There are many negative features that characterise this section of our population. It suffers from a high level of unemployment. Many among its ranks are uneducated and unskilled. It suffers from widespread and entrenched poverty. It is therefore victim to the entire spectrum of diseases of poverty and underdevelopment, including those associated with immune deficiency.'

23. An illuminating discussion of the history of ideas in disease management: Peter Baldwin, *Contagion and the State in Europe 1830-1930* (1999).

CHAPTER FIVE

1. President Mandela's address in Davos, Switzerland, in February 1997 is available on the UNAIDS website at www.unaids.org as well as at http://www.anc.org.za/ancdocs/ history/mandela/1997/sp970203.html.

2. The story of Ruth Mompati's remarks about gays in South Africa and their repudiation by Thabo Mbeki is told in Mark Gevisser and Edwin Cameron: *Defiant Desire – Gay and Lesbian Lives in South Africa* (Ravan Press, 1994 and Routledge, 1995) pp. 70, 75, 270.

3. *David John Cadwell Irving v Penguin Books Ltd and Deborah E Lipstadt* [2000] EWHC QB 115 (unreported judgment of Gray, J, Queens Bench Division, available at www.bailii.org/ ew/cases/EWHC/QB/2000/115.html).

4. My talk to the English Bar in London, September 2002, is published in (2003) 120 *South African Law Journal* 1.

5. On Holocaust denialism, see DD Guttenplan's account of the *Irving* v *Lipstadt* trial in DD Guttenplan, *The Holocaust on Trial* (Granta, 2001), and Michael Shermer & Alex Grobman,

Denying History: Who Says the Holocaust Never Happened and Why Do They Say It? (University of California Press, 2000).

6. The Edward A Smith Annual Lecture at Harvard Law School, 8 April 2003, is published in (2003) 120 *South African Law Journal* 525.

7. *Mail & Guardian* report on my Harvard lecture: *Mail & Guardian*, Johannesburg, Easter Thursday, 17 April 2003, 'Top Judge Slates Government's Dead Hand of Denialism', http://ww2.aegis.org/news/dmg/2003/MG030410.html.

8. Reports on Dr Roberto Giraldo's alleged association with the Health Department: 'Can SA afford Manto, asks DA', *iafrica.com*, 10 January 2003, available at www.iafrica.com/news/sa/200263.htm [5 June 2003]; S'Thembiso Msomi and Ranjeni Munusamy 'Manto wants Aids dissident as adviser', *Sunday Times*, 9 March 2003, available at www.sundaytimes.co.za/2003/03/09/news/news01.asp [5 June 2003]; 'Aids dissident "will not be adviser"', Thursday 13 March 2003, available at www.sundaytimes.co.za/zones/sundaytimes/newsst/newsst1047282629.asp [5 June 2003].

9. For reporting on alleged comments by the Minister of Finance see 'Manuel says AIDS drugs are "a lot of voodoo" ' *Business Day*, 19 March 2003. The headline was retracted, but the substance of the report was reasserted in 'The Thick End of the Wedge – Editor's Notebook', *Business Day*, 24 March 2003. See too Gill Moodie, 'More flak for Manuel over AIDS comments', *Sunday Times,* 23 March 2003.

10. The 'assumption' that HIV causes AIDS: 'So Many Questions', interview by Chris Barron with the minister in the office of the president, Essop Pahad, *Sunday Times*, 15 September 2002.

11. The 'premise' that HIV causes AIDS: government advertisement: 'Let's Build a People's Contract to Fight HIV/AIDS!', Johannesburg *Sunday Times*, 23 March 2003, incisively analysed by Timothy Trengove Jones, 'Add pinch of salt to state advert on its AIDS policy', Johannesburg *Business Day*, 1 April 2003.

12. For AIDS mortality statistics in South Africa, see Debbie Bradshaw et al, 'Initial Estimates from the South African National Burden of Disease Study, 2000', Medical Research Council Policy Brief, No 1, March 2003, available at www.mrc.ac.za/bod/bod.htm [accessed 17 June 2003]. This report emphasises that HIV/AIDS is the leading cause of death amongst young adults of both genders, and is expected to continue to grow rapidly 'unless interventions that reduce mortality and morbidity become widely available'. In graphic terms, that 'without interventions aimed at reducing HIV/AIDS mortality, HIV/AIDS will [by 2010] *more than double the burden of premature mortality* (YLLs [- years of life lost]) experienced in 2000'.

13. For stop/start progress in 2002/2003 in devising a national treatment plan, see Government Communication and Information Service, *Update on the National HIV and AIDS Programme* (19 March 2003), available at www.gov.za/issues/HIV/update19-mar03full.htm [17 June 2003]; Department of Labour *Statement on the NEDLAC HIV/AIDS Task Team by Adv. Rams Ramashia* (19 March 2003), available at www.gov.za/issues/HIV/index.html [17 June 2003]; 'Nedlac to broach HIV/Aids plan', *Sunday Times*, 23 February 2003.

14. Zackie Achmat's comments on AIDS policies as a 'holocaust against the poor': Speech at the centenary reunion of the Rhodes Trust at University of Cape Town on Saturday 1 February 2003; University of Natal graduation Saturday 5 April 2003.

15. For UNAIDS estimates, see UNAIDS *Report on the Global HIV/AIDS epidemic 2002* at 45:

'In the 45 most affected countries, it is projected that between 2000 and 2020, 68 million people will die earlier than they would have in the absence of AIDS.'

16. Eric Miyeni Talkshow, SAfm, 14h30 on Thursday, 24 April 2003.

17. The case of the women murderers: *S v Sopronia Aloma van Heerden and Bernadette Laus*, 274/2002, judgment of 19 May 2003 (unreported).

18. The case of the magistrate and the doctor seeking bail: *Magistrate, Stutterheim v Mashiya* 2004 (5) SA 209 (SCA), 2003 (2) SACR 106 (SCA).

19. Justice Minister Penuell Maduna's attack on me for allegedly comparing the government's AIDS policies with the Jewish genocide and with 'Hitler' reported by Christi van der Westhuizen in Johannesburg *Beeld* and Bloemfontein *Volksblad*, 4 June 2003, and by John Battersby, Farhana Ismail and André Koopman in *Sunday Independent*, 15 June 2003.

20. On the United States controversy about judicial 'free speech' and participation by judges in current political controversy, see *Republican Party of Minnesota v Suzanne White*, 536 US 765 (2002) (clause prohibiting candidates for election as judges from expressing their 'views on disputed legal or political issues' declared by 5-4 majority of court to violate free speech guarantees of first amendment of United States Constitution). See also Ronald Dworkin's debate with Judge Richard Posner, R Dworkin, 'Philosophy and Monica Lewinsky', *The New York Review of Books* 25, May 2000, pp. 48-64.

21. Excerpt from the final report of the Truth and Reconciliation Commission, October 1998, vol. 5, chapter 6, para.158, pp. 253-254.

22. An illuminating Australian perspective on the question whether judges should or may speak out about matters of current political moment is contained in the article by Justice McMurdo, President, Court of Appeal, Supreme Court of Queensland, 'Taking Judges at Their Word', *The Canberra Times*, 22 October 2001, available at http://canberra.yourguide.com.au/detail.asp?story_id=99769&y=2001&m=10&class, [accessed 16 July 2004].

23. Chief Justice Arthur Chaskalson's Bram Fischer Memorial Lecture, 'Human Dignity as a Foundational Value of our Constitutional Order', is published in (2000) 16, *South African Journal on Human Rights* 193-205. The quotation in the text appears on page 205.

24. Carmel Rickard's report on South African judges' statements on the Zimbabwe rule of law crisis, 'SA judges throw the book at Mugabe', Johannesburg *Sunday Times*, 4 March 2004, is available at http://www.suntimes.co.za/2001/03/04/news/news03.htm, [accessed 14 July 2004].

25. President Mbeki's State of the Nation address at the opening of the new Parliament on Friday 21 May 2004 is available at http://www.info.gov.za/search97cgi/s97_cgi?action=View&VdkVgwKey=%2E%2E%.

26. Constitution of the Republic of South Africa, section 174(6): 'The President must appoint the judges of all other courts on the advice of the Judicial Service Commission.'

CHAPTER SIX

1. Christopher Moraka's story told by Siphokazi Mthathi 'Christopher Moraka (1956-2000)' at http://www.tac.org.za/Documents/Statements/chris.htm [accessed 22 May 2004].

2. Definition of 'patent' from Concise Oxford Dictionary.

3. Information on origin of patents from *Encyclopaedia Britannica*, 1978, 15th Edition, Macropaedia vol. 13, p. 1071. Patent office claim on Patent Office website, http://www.patent.gov.uk/patent/history/fivehundred/origins.htm, [accessed 31 May 2004].

4. The oath of office that judges take under South Africa's Constitution is contained in Schedule Two, Item 6 of the Constitution.

5. Interpretation of TRIPS draws on Correa, C, 2002, 'Implications of the Doha Declaration on the TRIPS Agreement and Public Health', World Health Organisation, Health Economics and Drugs EDM Series no. 12, p. i.

6. Discussion of patent rights adapted from Jonathan Berger, thesis, *Tripping Over Patents*, drawing on David Vaver, 'Intellectual Property Today: Of Myths and Paradoxes' (1990) 69 *Canadian Bar Review* 98 at 126; Christopher May, *A Global Political Economy of Intellectual Property Rights: The new enclosures?* (London: Routledge, 2000) at 49; Robert Weissman, 'A Long, Strange TRIPS: The Pharmaceutical Industry Drive to Harmonize Global Intellectual Property Rules, and the Remaining Legal Alternatives Available to Third World Countries' (1996) 17, *University of Pennsylvania Journal of International Economic Law* 1069 at 1087; and Edwin Cameron and Jonathan Berger, 'Patents, and Public Health: Principle, Politics and Paradox', British Academy Lecture in Law, Edinburgh 19 October 2004, forthcoming in the *Proceedings of the British Academy*.

7. A South African case that expresses the public benefit theory of patent exclusivity is *Syntheta (Pty) Ltd (formerly Delta G Scientific (Pty) Ltd v Janssen Pharmaceutica NV and Another*, 1999 (1) South African Law Reports 85 (Supreme Court of Appeal) at 88I-J: '[I]t is part of the theory upon which our patent law is based that the limited statutory monopoly afforded a patentee is seen as a means of encouraging inventors to put their inventions into practice because by this means they obtain the financial rewards their inventive gifts warrant. But what perhaps requires more emphasis . . . is that, by encouraging inventors to put their inventions to use, the benefit to the public (an essential quid pro quo of the theory) is served.'

8. On the contretemps between Ghana and Glaxo Wellcome PLC, *Wall Street Journal* writer Mark Schoofs wrote on 1 December 2000: 'In the midst of the wrenching international debate over how to get expensive HIV drugs into Africa, pharmaceutical giant Glaxo Wellcome PLC has set off a new controversy by trying to block access to less-costly generic versions of its top-selling AIDS medicine. In letters to a drug distributor in Ghana and an Indian generic-drug maker, Glaxo said sales of generic versions of its drug, Combivir, in Ghana would be illegal because they would be violating company patents. As a result, the Indian company, Cipla Ltd of Bombay, has stopped selling its low-cost version in Ghana, a small country in west Africa. However, officials at the multilateral African agency that issued the Glaxo patents in question said they are either invalid in Ghana or don't apply. Glaxo's actions are "wrong," said Christopher Kiige, head patent examiner of the African Regional Industrial Property Organization. He says: "If [Glaxo officials] went to court they would lose." A Glaxo spokesman in London says the drug maker believes its drug is patent-protected in Ghana but declined to provide an explanation or legal documentation.' Source: http://www.mindfully.org/Industry/Glaxo-Ghana-AIDS-Drugs.htm, citing Mark Schoofs, *Wall Street Journal*, 1 Dec 2000.

9. The claim that it takes USD$800 million to develop a new drug: Tufts University Study authored by Joseph DiMasi, December 2001, http://www.biohope.org/media/article.cfm?articleid=2130&state=na.

10. For drug company profits, see Marcia Angell, 'The Truth About the Drug Companies', *New York Review of Books*, 15 July 2004, pp. 52-58. Tina Rosenberg of the *New York Times* has written powerful articles on patents and public health, including 'Look at Brazil', *New York Times*, January 28, 2001.

11. For sub-Saharan Africa accounting for just over 1% of global pharmaceutical sales, see 'Drugs: Round One to Africa', by Nick Mathiason, London *Observer*, 22 April 2001, http://www.guardian.co.uk/Archive/Article/0,4273,4173653,00.html.

12. On the injustices of the world trade system and patent enforcement, see the Oxfam paper, 'Patent Injustice – How World Trade Rules Threaten the Health of Poor People', http://www.maketradefair.com/en/index.php?file=05092003160059.htm&cat=2&subcat=7&select=5.

13. Nathan Geffen, 'Pharmaceutical Patents, Human Rights and the HIV/AIDS Epidemic', paper presented on 22 May 2001 to the World Business Council on Sustainable Development.

14. Absence of patent protection spurs nineteenth century invention: Petra Moser, of the Massachusetts Institute of Technology's Sloan School of Management, PhD, see NBER Working Papers by Petra Moser: 'How Do Patent Laws Influence Innovation? Evidence from Nineteenth-Century World Fairs' August 2003, located at http://www.nber.org/papers/w9909.

15. The United States has itself not always protected intellectual property – to its own historical benefit in the nineteenth century. See Steve Lohr: 'On intellectual property, U.S. forgets its own past', *New York Times*, 16 October 2002.

16. For United States profiting from copying English inventions: from 'A Stroll Through Patent History', by Teresa Riordan, *New York Times*, 29 September 2003.

17. The argument that poverty and not patents is the problem is made by J Shikwati, 'Poverty, not patents, is to blame', Johannesburg *Business Day*, 1 June 2004, controverted by Jonathan Berger, and Nathan Geffen, 'Patent Nonsense', Johannesburg *Business Day*, 14 June 2004.

18. See the AFP, 'Poverty Hinders Zimbabwe AIDS Battle' Johannesburg *Business Day*, http://www.bday.co.za/bday/content/direct/1,3523,1639808-6078-0,00.html [accessed 16 June 2004].

19. For the estimated 40 million people living with HIV/AIDS globally, of whom approximately 95 per cent live in developing countries, and the fact that only 8 per cent of these have access to antiretroviral treatment, see 'Treating 3 million by 2005: Making it happen – the WHO strategy' (World Health Organization: Geneva, 2003) at 3 and 4-5.

20. Information on Brazilians on antiretroviral treatment from UNAIDS Report on the Global Epidemic, 2004, http://www.unaids.org/bangkok2004/GAR2004_html/GAR2004_26_en.htm#TopOfPage. Further information on Brazil from UNAIDS, *The Brazilian Response to HIV/AIDS. Best Practices,* Brazilian Ministry of Health, Secretariat for Health Policies, National Co-ordination for STD and AIDS, ed. by Ermenegyldo Munhoz, Jr, 2000.

21. Brazil's governmental action brings lower drug prices: see 'Brazil, Merck Negotiate 25% Price Discount on Antiretroviral Drug Efavirenz', kaisernetwork.org, 19/2/2003, http://www.kaisernetwork.org/daily_reports/rep_index.cfm?hint=1&DR_ID=20928 [accessed 13 June 2004].

22. South African Constitutional Court on necessity for coordinated government/civil society cooperation: *Minister of Health* v *Treatment Action Campaign (No 2)* 2002 (5) South African Law Reports 721 (CC) paras 123, 125 and 126.

23. BMS Thailand move in 2004: Statement by Dianne Jones of BMS's regional office in Singapore, quoted in *The Nation*, 17 January 2004; 'US giant gives up right to AIDS pill', by Mukdawan Sakboon, and 'Prices to fall, NGOs must withdraw suits', by Apaluck Bhatiasevi in *The Bangkok Post*, 17 January 2004.

24. Competition Act 89 of 1998 section 2(b) – the purpose of the legislation is 'to provide consumers with competitive prices and product choices'. The Competition Commission was established under section 19 and has the power to investigate and evaluate contraventions (section 21(1)(c)) and to negotiate and conclude consent orders (section 21(1)(f) regarding complaints about prohibited practices.
25. Boehringer Ingelheim's offer of free nevirapine to poor countries wishing to inhibit perinatal transmission of HIV on 7 July 2000: http://www.hivandhepatitis.com/recent/perinatal/070700.html.
26. Dean Baker and Nonko Chatani of the Centre for Economic and Policy Research: Baker, D, 2001, 'The High Cost of Protectionism: The Case of Intellectual Property Claims'.
27. South African activists suggesting patent system innovations: Nathan Geffen and Jonathan Berger, 'Patent System for Medicines Needs to be Revamped', Johannesburg *This-Day*, 26 January 2004.
28. Senior drug company executive on profits and the Red Cross: Pfizer executive vice president, CL Clemente, quoted in 'Companies fear precedent as they cut AIDS drug prices for Africa', Theresa Agovino, Associated Press, 20 April 2001.

CHAPTER SEVEN

1. Testimony of Nontsikelelo Zwedala before South Africa Competition Commission in the case of *Hazel Tau v GlaxoSmithKline and Boehringer Ingelheim* quoted in Mkhutyukelwa, B, Mtonjeni, T, and Jacobs, V, 'David Patient Knows Nothing About Africans Living in Poverty', http://www.tac.org.za/newsletter/2002/ns21_10_2002.txt, [accessed 23 May 2004].
2. Disruption of Vice-President Albert J Gore's presidential campaign launch on 16 June 1999: Behrman, Greg, *The Invisible People* (Free Press, 2004) p.141.
3. Information on success of MSF's Khayelitsha antiretroviral project from IRIN Plus News, circulated on AF-AIDS email list on 4 June 2003, marked 'copyright UN Office for the Coordination of Humanitarian Affairs'.
4. 2001 insert in Johannesburg *Sunday Times* expressing scepticism about practicability of large-scale treatment access programmes: LoveLife, 2001, 'Impending Catastrophe Revisited: an update on the HIV/AIDS epidemic in South Africa', published as a supplement to the *Sunday Times*, June 2001, Henry J Kaiser Family Foundation.
5. Health writers continuing to contend that prevention is more cost-effective than treatment: See Marseille, E, Hofman, P, and J. Kahn, 'HIV Prevention before HAART in Southern Africa', *The Lancet*, vol. 359, May 25 2002.
6. International Monetary Fund discussion paper: Haacker, M, *Providing Health Care to HIV Patients in Southern Africa. IMF Policy Discussion Paper PDP/01/3*. International Monetary Fund, 2001.
7. Professor Nicoli Nattrass, *The Moral Economy of AIDS in South Africa* (Cambridge University Press, 2004) pp. 36-55.
8. East African study on cost-effectiveness: Sweat M, Gregorich S, Sangiwa G, Furlonge C, Balmer D, Kamenga C, Grinstead O, Coates T, 'Cost-effectiveness of voluntary HIV-1 counselling and testing in reducing sexual transmission of HIV-1 in Kenya and Tanzania', *The Lancet* vol. 356 (2000), pp. 113 – 121.
9. Costing study showing that efficacy of non-treatment HIV interventions is limited: Nathan Geffen, Nicoli Nattrass and Chris Raubenheimer, 'The Cost of HIV Prevention

and Treatment Interventions in South Africa', CSSR Working Paper No. 28, University of Cape Town, January 2003.

10. Wartime 'triage' decision-making applied to prevention/care decisions in AIDS epidemic interventions: Creese A, Floyd K, Alban A, Guinness L, 'Cost-effectiveness of HIV/AIDS interventions in Africa: a systematic review of the evidence' *The Lancet*, vol. 359, 25 May 2002, 1635-1642.

11. Is treatment for AIDS a right if people with AIDS are responsible for their own condition? Benatar D, 'HIV and the Hemi-Nanny State', *The Lancet Infectious Diseases* 2002; 2:394.

12. Paul Farmer on arguments against the poor: Farmer P, *Pathologies of Power: Health, Human Rights and the New War on the Poor* (University of California Press, 2003).

13. USAID director Andrew Natsios on poor Africans' time-keeping abilities: Bob Herbert, 'Refusing to save Africans', *New York Times* 12 June 2001.

14. Health Minister Tshabalala-Msimang's comments on poor Africans' watches: 'AIDS fund poses worldwide challenge', by Laurie Garrett, *Newsday* staff writer, June 17, 2001: http://www.newsday.com/news/health/ny-aids20-aids061701.story.

15. In June 2002 there were apparently June 2002 13 814 million South African users of mobile telephones: see http://www.cia.gov/cia/publications/factbook/geos/sf.html#Comm. The figure for mid-2004 was 14.4 million, and it is projected that in 2006 there will be 19 million: Vodacom statistics http://www.cellular.co.za/stats/statistics_south_africa.htm.

16. Africans' 'toilet / outhouse / bush / tree': David Patient, Wednesday 18 Sep 2002, 'All pigs fed and ready to fly!!' http://archives.hst.org.za/af-aids/msg00523.html, [accessed 23 May 2004]; rebutted by Mkhutyukelwa B, Mtonjeni T, and Jacobs V, 2002, 'David Patient Knows Nothing About Africans Living in Poverty', http://www.tac.org.za/newsletter/2002/ns21_10_2002.txt, [23 May 2004].

17. Somerset Hospital study showing excellent adherence by poor township residents: Orrell C, Bangsberg DR, Badri M, Wood R, 'Adherence is not a barrier to successful antiretroviral therapy in South Africa', *AIDS* 2003 June 13; 17(9): 1369-75.

18. John Kenneth Galbraith, quote from JK Galbraith, *The World Economy since the Wars* (Mandarin, 1994).

19. Concluding quotation from Paul Farmer, Preface to the paperback edition of *Infections and Inequalities* (University of California Press, revised edition 2000) p. xxviii.

CHAPTER EIGHT

1. The practical project of providing antiretroviral treatment to those needing it as 'the most extensive humanitarian venture in human history': Laurie Garrett, 'Bragging in Bangkok' *New York Times* 16 July 2004.

2. On the 'unspeakability' of AIDS in South Africa, given the period of denialism, see Debbie Posel, 'Democracy in a Time of AIDS', *Wiser Review*, no.1, July 2004.

Notes

Index of Persons

Acknowledgements

This book would not have been written without the generous support and commitment and sustaining interest of many friends and colleagues. Hannes van Zyl, then managing director of Tafelberg/NB Publishers, instigated it all. He heard me speak at the Durban 2000 AIDS conference, and contacted me afterwards to say that I 'had to' write a book about my experiences in the epidemic. Yes, yes. Some day. Well, Hannes was not to be fobbed off. He phoned and visited an followed up and exhorted and envisioned and enjoined. The book's realisation is due to his pivotal encouragement. Although Hannes later left formal publishing, he read and improved the text, and helped Erika Oosthuysen, my publisher, to whom I also express grateful thanks, to shepherd the book to production.

I owe much to friends and colleagues who read and commented on the draft text or parts of it: Carole H Lewis, Mark Behr, Gilbert J Marcus, Jonathan Lewis, Robert Wintemute, Sappho Dias, Anthony Hamburger, Robert W Nugent, Zelda Kruger, Zingi Mkefa, Zackie Achmat, Andrew Park, Derek Bodell and Lorraine Chaskalson. And of course the Richters, all of whom read every word and made many improvements. And to Wim Richter, thanks for his wizardry and effort with the photographs.

In July 2004, at a stage critical to completion, Samar Ali, a student from Vanderbilt University Law School, Nashville, Tennessee, breezed into my life off the trans-Atlantic flight in a gust of energy and good will. Through her contacts with the family of Archbishop Emeritus Desmond Tutu she had sought a legal internship in South Africa. So she came to me for five creative, affirming, energetic weeks – generally improving the climate and the country and the world, but also doing an immense amount of minute checking and researching and following up. She also read the text and made innumerable useful suggestions.

Special thanks to Mark Behr for consistent encouragement and faith, especially for his sobering conviction that the book could be better than it is. And special thanks to Madeleine Kuhn, Zelda Kruger and Karen Hurt, for translating their faith in the book into always-generous encouragement.

I was able to start writing during eleven weeks of sabbatical leave in the northern autumn of 2003 as a visiting fellow at All Souls College, Oxford. I am indebted to the Warden, Dr John Davis, and the Fellows, for a wonderful stay. And to the Kaiser Family Foundation for generously converting the academic benefits connected with the 2000 Nelson Mandela Health and Human Rights Award (normally to be taken up in the United States) into monetary support for my stay in Oxford.

My debt to Nathan Geffen is particularly big. He willingly supplied two crucial draft chapters, on patents and sustainability of treatment in resource-poor settings – and with characteristic self-effacement sought to claim no credit. He also gave meticulously truthful and rigorous commentary on the whole text.

I am greatly indebted to Professor Jakes Gerwel and to Shaun Johnson for immeasurably enhancing the book. Shaun also read the manuscript and suggested one indispensable addition.

EDWIN CAMERON
Brixton, Johannesburg
3 February 2005

Edwin Cameron studied at Stellenbosch, Oxford and the University of South Africa, winning top academic honours at all three universities. He joined the Johannesburg Bar in 1983, and from 1986 practised as a human rights lawyer at the University of the Witwatersrand's Centre for Applied Legal Studies (CALS), where in 1989 he was awarded a personal professorship in law. While at CALS, he co-drafted the Charter of Rights on AIDS and HIV, co-founded the AIDS Consortium and founded and was the first director of the AIDS Law Project.

In October 1994 President Mandela appointed him an Acting Judge of the High Court to chair a Commission into illegal arms deals. He was appointed permanently to the High Court in 1995. In 1999/2000 he served for a year as an Acting Justice in the Constitutional Court before being appointed to the Supreme Court of Appeal.

Since 1998, he has chaired the Council of the University of the Witwatersrand. He is the Patron of the Guild Cottage Children's Home, of the Soweto HIV/AIDS Counsellors' Association (SOHACA) and of Community AIDS Response (CARE).

Edwin Cameron has co-authored a number of books, including *Defiant Desire – Gay and Lesbian Lives in South Africa* and *Honoré's South African Law of Trusts*.

He has received many awards and distinctions. These include Honorary Fellowships of Keble College, Oxford and of the Society for Advanced Legal Studies, London; the Nelson Mandela Award for Health and Human Rights (2000); Stellenbosch University's Alumnus Award (2000), Transnet's HIV/AIDS Champions Award and the San Francisco AIDS Foundation Excellence in Leadership Award (2003). In 2002 the Bar of England and Wales honoured him with a Special Award for his contribution to international jurisprudence and the protection of human rights.